To

Mary

my wife, my partner, my companion, my colleague, my friend

STEVEN A. COLE

To my wife

Averil Michelle Leimon

whose positive and empathic approach to therapeutic work has contributed so much to my own ideas and whose tolerance and support have made my contribution to this book possible.

JULIAN BIRD

CONTRIBUTORS

THOMAS L. CAMPBELL, MD
Co-editor, Families, Systems & Health
Professor of Family Medicine and Psychiatry
University of Rochester School of Medicine and Dentistry
Rochester, New York

CECILE A. CARSON, MD
Clinical Associate Professor of Medicine & Psychiatry
University of Rochester Medical Center
Rochester, New York

KATHY COLE-KELLY, MSW, MS
Associate Professor of Family Medicine
Case Western Reserve University School of Medicine
Metrohealth Medical Center
Cleveland, Ohio

GEOFFREY H. GORDON, MD, FACP
Associate Director, Clinical Education and Research
Bayer Institute for Health Care Communication
Milford, Connecticut

DENNIS H. NOVACK, MD
Professor of Medicine
Associate Dean of Medical Education
MCP Hahnemann University
Philadelphia, Pennsylvania

DAVID J. STEELE, PhD
Associate Professor of Family Medicine
Director, Integrated Clinical Experience Program
University of Nebraska Medical Center
Omaha, Nebraska

FOREWORD to the Second Edition

Over 20 years ago, I had my first experience in medical interviewing as part of a second-year medical school course on physical diagnosis. I was videotaped while interviewing an elderly gentleman on the inpatient service. I was terrified as our group of students reviewed my videotape with a consulting psychiatrist. Each utterance and gesture was analyzed in great detail. At that time there were no textbooks on interviewing for medical students. We learned through trial and error. What I would have done for a copy of *The Medical Interview: The Three-Function Approach* to help guide me through the process of learning communication skills.

The teaching of communication skills in medical schools and residencies has improved dramatically over the past two decades. Nearly every U.S. medical school now has a required interviewing course. There are several basic texts on teaching and learning medical interviewing, but none present as simple and clear a model as *The Three-Function Approach.* Communicating effectively with patients is a complex and challenging task that calls for a conceptually clear and easily understandable approach. Long checklists of tasks to be accomplished during the medical interview can be overwhelming to the learner and even the experienced clinician.

Currently, I teach communication skills to medical students and family medicine residents, and I have found the three-function approach to be very useful. During each teaching session, we can focus on a different function and practice the component skills. When I am directly observing a resident in the clinic or reviewing a videotape, the three-function approach provides a helpful framework for feedback. ("Jim, you did a nice job building a relationship with this patient [function 1] and thoroughly assessing her problems [function 2]. Let's talk about how you can negotiate a treatment plan more effectively with her [function 3])." I can then review the specific skills that are a part of the third function.

The first edition of this text was a major contribution to the field and has been adopted by over 20 U.S. medical schools. This second updated edition represents a significant advance and a modest expansion of its predecessor. The text has been completely rewritten and 12 chapters are brand new. I am particularly pleased with the reordering of the functions, so that "building the relationship" with the patient comes first and foremost, before gathering data or assessing the problem. This change recognizes that the quality of the interview depends upon establishing rapport and developing a therapeutic relationship with the patient. There is also a clearer linkage between the three functions and each step or phase of the interview. These changes will be very helpful for medical students and residents learning communication skills.

This second edition offers much for the more experienced student or clinician. There are eight chapters on common communication challenges, including interviewing elderly patients, dealing with sexual issues, overcoming language and cultural issues, and four chapters on more advanced communication skills. This text provides a framework for a very rich course on communication skills for medical students or residents. It will be useful for training other clinicians as well, especially nurse practitioners, physician assistants and social workers, and for continuing medical education.

Over 30 years ago, George Engel first challenged biomedicine to be more scientific and include psychosocial data as part of the clinical process. He wrote

> The dominant model of disease today is biomedical, with molecular biology its basic scientific discipline. It assumes disease to be fully accounted for by deviations from the norm of measurable biological (somatic) variables. It leaves no room within its framework for the social, psychological, and behavioral dimensions of illness.[1]

He further argued that

> the existing biomedical model does not suffice. To provide a basis for understanding the determinants of disease and arriving at rational treatments and patterns of health care, a medical model must also take into account the patient, the social context in which he lives and the complementary system devised by society to deal with the disruptive effects of illness, that is, the physician role and the health care system. This requires a biopsychosocial model.[1]

Engel contended that the biopsychosocial model represented a more scientific approach to health care.

Since the publication of his seminal article, the biopsychosocial model has been widely accepted in medicine, especially in primary care. A large body of research supporting connections between psychosocial and biomedical processes has been published, most notably in the field of psychoimmunology. With the spread of the biopsychosocial model, there has been a growing interest in the doctor-patient relationship and communication skills.

Until recently, medical interviewing was considered an art, the skills of which were discovered by observing other practitioners and practiced with one's own patients. There was little science in medical interviewing, and no clear support for specific skills to teach. Beginning with the pio-

---

[1] Engel G: The need for a new medical model: a challenge for biomedicine, *Science* 196:129-136, 1977.

neering work of pediatrician Barbara Korsch, research on medical interviewing has burgeoned, and an evidence-based approach to teaching communication is now possible. A large body of research clearly establishes that physician-patient communication affects a broad range of health outcomes, including patients' satisfaction, adherence, physical and mental health, and risk of malpractice suits.

There is also a growing body of research on how to teach the medical interview. Teaching communication skills should be skill based (versus attitudinal) and experiential (versus observational) and occur in small groups or one on one. Essential ingredients include systematic delineation and definition of the necessary skills, observation of these skills, constructive and detailed feedback by the instructor, and rehearsal and practice of the skills. Unfortunately, this process takes an enormous amount of faculty time, and there are not enough trained faculty to do this teaching. A major challenge for the next decade is to expand faculty development programs to train faculty in how to teach medical interviewing skills.

One of the most important steps for improving communication skills in medicine is to include the assessment of these skills in medical school and certifying examinations. Students put the most effort into learning those areas of knowledge and skills that will appear on these exams. The three-function approach provides a framework for developing clinical examinations. Family practice in Canada has considerable experience with this type of examination. For almost a decade the College of Family Physicians of Canada has used simulated patient-evaluators in its certifying examinations to assess candidates' communication skills. The National Board of Medical Examiners and some of the specialty boards are making plans to include Objective, Standardized Clinical Evaluations (OSCE) as part of their examinations and to assess communication skills. When the National Board includes the assessment of communication skills, we can expect an accelerated interest in teaching interviewing to medical students. Every medical student will have to demonstrate proficiency in communication skills before obtaining a medical license, and every medical school will receive a "report card" on how well their students do on the communication section of the National Boards. This will lead to more emphasis on interviewing throughout medical school training and an increased demand for books like this one. When interviewing skills are considered as important as medical knowledge and physical examination skills, and proficiency in interviewing must be demonstrated for licensure and board certification, we will see more widespread implementation of the biopsychosocial model and more effective and compassionate medical care.

Thomas L. Campbell, MD
Professor of Family Medicine and Psychiatry
University of Rochester School of Medicine and Dentistry
Chair, Advisory Council, Bayer Institute for Health Care Communication

FOREWORD to the First Edition

IMPORTANCE OF THE INTERVIEW

The medical interview is the most important clinical tool available to health practitioners. This is so for many reasons, both personal and professional.

On the personal level, the interview is the task in medicine one will do the most often and spend the most time on. An average primary care practitioner may do between 120,000 and 160,000 interviews in a professional lifetime of 40 years. Therefore, it is worth doing expertly and cogently.

Professionally, the interview is the major medium of care. It determines the problems addressed and helped. It forms the doctor-patient relationship so central to the satisfaction of both practitioner and patient. It determines one's knowledge of the life context of the illness which may hold the secrets of etiology and healing. It is the medium of patient education about the illness, the diagnostic process, and the therapy. For all these reasons, the interview is well worth the attention of practitioners at every level, throughout a professional lifetime.

THE INTERVIEW IS KNOWABLE

Twenty years ago, the interview was the subject of charisma and speculation. Teaching was based on the precept that students should do as the teachers do. Teachers were often from a clinical faculty or chosen on the basis of self-assertion or charismatic appeal. This all changed with the advent of fast, economical videotaping of interviews. Barbara Korsch and her colleagues ushered in the scientific era of interview study with her classic studies of pediatricians and their patients and mothers in the emergency department and clinic. In these studies, a camera was placed unobtrusively in the corner of the ceiling of examining rooms and, with permission, the encounters were taped. It turned out that pediatricians and their patients were speaking significantly different languages, not understanding one another and therefore talking at cross purposes.

Since then, thousands of articles have looked at the content, process, outcomes, and correlates of interviews and interviewers. A recent bibliography, attempting to highlight the leading papers in the field, identified

125 papers and books, and the Task Force on the Doctor and Patient has over 600 articles in its core files. Thus, the medical interview is a subject about which specific, empirical knowledge exists. It is the responsibility of each diligent clinician or future clinician to know at least the main points of this literature.

THE INTERVIEW IS MASTERABLE

Nor is this simply an academic issue. If one has a 10 percent inefficiency in one's interviewing, one will lose over 2 years of practice time as a result. If one fails to identify one of the three problems the average patient has in mind during a typical visit, one will overlook over 100,000 problems over a professional lifetime!

Nor is the interview a matter solely of talent. A variety of authors, in the United States, the Netherlands, and in the United Kingdom have shown that simple efforts to improve interviewing skills will succeed. In one experiment, a single interview practice course of six sessions led to durable improvements that were still measurable after 6 years. Although there is always room for improvement, the reading of a text such as this accompanied by appropriate exercises can be expected to lead to significantly enhanced mastery of the basics of effective interviewing.

The opposite is equally true. Those interviewing without adequate training and supervision are likely to make one or more serious errors regularly. These may have detrimental effects on diagnostic ability, practitioner satisfaction, and patient satisfaction and compliance.

THE INTERVIEW HAS STRUCTURE AND FUNCTIONS

Learning about the interview has been enhanced by several conceptual advances in the recent past. The first of these is the recognition that the interview has structure and it has functions. The structure may be viewed simply as beginning, middle and end, or complexly with up to ten structural elements. Each of these encompasses a series of specific concerns and behaviors which if mastered lead to better results.

Likewise, the interview has functions. Julian Bird and Steven Cole have led in the definition of a three-function model of the interview which has enormous heuristic utility in learning about interviewing. The three functions get expressed variously but the formulation in this book is both authoritative and especially clear. The three functions, like the structural elements, have specific skills underlying their execution that can and must be learned, practiced, and mastered. While the advanced learner may eventually move to a more complex view of the functions of the interview, the three-function model is the place to start.

PRACTICE, CURIOSITY, FEEDBACK

Several approaches will enhance the learning of the material covered so succinctly here in this introductory text. The first is to attempt to practice often and with focused awareness of specific behaviorally defined learning goals. One's chances of accomplishing something are increased if one knows what that something is. Second, a sense of scientific curiosity and humanistic wonder will make the work more effective and more fun. The human drama is heightened by illness and we practitioners have the privilege of front row seats. Our patients share with us most of the wisdom and understanding to be obtained in life and we are in a wonderful position to learn from them and their experience. Finally, obtaining direct feedback about one's performance through self review and review with a skilled tutor will increase the breadth and depth of possible learning since it will be less handicapped by one's own blind spots.

Practice with curiosity and feedback can convert a scary process into a lively challenge.

THIS BOOK

Dr. Cole has created a brief, conceptually clear, clinically relevant beginning text ideally suited for beginning students of the practitioner's arts. The book is organized along the lines of the three-function model making the steps to mastery explicit, understandable and discrete.

But there is much here also for the experienced clinician who is new to the study of the interview. Dr. Cole has quietly incorporated a superb synthesis of the literature suitable as a reintroduction this now robust field of inquiry and practice.

For this and for his many significant contributions to the substance of the field, I and my colleagues in the study of the interview salute and thank Dr. Cole and congratulate those students who decide to embark on this short journey of learning and discovery with him. This is a fine way to inaugurate a lifetime of practice and learning about this fine core clinical skill.

Mack Lipkin, Jr., MD

Associate Professor of Medicine
Director, Primary Care Medicine
New York University School of Medicine
New York, New York
Codirector, Task Force on the Doctor and Patient for the Society of General Internal Medicine (SGIM)

PREFACE

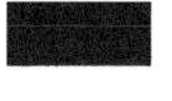

WHY CREATE A NEW EDITION OF THIS STUDENT TEXTBOOK ON THE MEDICAL INTERVIEW?

Since its publication in 1991, this text has become an important component in the communication skills training of many student physicians in the United States and abroad. Many U.S. medical schools have adopted the book, and the three-function model has become the conceptual basis of their courses on medical interviewing. The book's approach to the learning of interviewing—linking skills to functions—is also widely used throughout Europe, Canada, and Latin America. Feedback we have received from colleagues, instructors, and students has been very positive and gratifying.

Since original publication of the book, however, we have also received many excellent suggestions for revisions and expansions from numerous sources. In addition, our understanding of the dynamics of efficient and effective interviewing has deepened as a result of recent research findings, theoretical contributions, and clinical experience. Finally, reflection on our own teaching experiences has broadened our understanding of the learning process. Together, these factors demanded a second edition of our text.

Overall, the most important conceptual and pragmatic advance concerns a fundamental change in sequencing of the three core functions of the interview. The first edition of the book placed primacy on the skills associated with gathering data. Rapport and relationship-building skills became the focus of the second function of the interview. This revised edition, in contrast, reverses the presentation of these two core functions, placing primacy on the functional importance of building the relationship. Without adequate rapport, the physician cannot understand or manage the patient's problem(s) effectively. Every effective interview must focus on the need to build the relationship from the very beginning and attend to this functional requirement throughout the entire communication process.

In addition to changing the sequence for presenting and learning function one and function two, the revised edition of the book articulates more concrete linkages between the structural components of the interview and the functions they serve. The first edition of the book presented each sequential structural element of the interview without a clearly stated relationship to the functions previously described. In contrast, this edition now makes more explicit connections between structure and function—i.e., between the eight basic structural elements of the interview (Chapters 7 to 14) and the three core interview functions.

The second edition is also considerably more comprehensive than the first edition. In response to readers' requests, we are including eight new chapters on communication challenges: sexual issues in the interview; interviewing the elderly patient; overcoming language and cultural barriers; family interviewing; troubling personality styles and somatization; nonadherence, lifestyle change, and stress; psychosis, delirium, and dementia; and breaking bad news.

Finally, the limited discussion of higher order skills in the first edition has been significantly enriched by four new chapters on nonverbal communication, use of the self in medical care, psychologic principles in the medical interview, and integration of structure and function. Throughout the revised text, all chapters have been updated to incorporate significant new research and theoretic advances of the last decade.

WHY USE THE "THREE-FUNCTION APPROACH" FOR LEARNING TO INTERVIEW?

Many other good introductory texts on interviewing are currently available. None of these, however, seem to provide beginners with what they need most—a cognitive framework that is simple enough to master relatively easily and quickly, yet robust enough to touch upon the most important dimensions of the communication process. Many texts seem to founder at one of the two extremes: some oversimplify complex processes, ignoring important aspects of interviewing, while others flood and confuse beginners with more information and clinical insights than can possibly be assimilated in limited periods of time.

This text presents an educational device, the three-function model of the medical interview, specifically designed to overcome these problems. First developed by Julian Bird, and later developed by Steven Cole and others, this model offers learners a simplified, straightforward approach to communication processes that is also rich enough to address many of the subtleties of interviewing at the same time.

The three functions address the three core objectives of the doctor-patient communication process: (1) building the relationship; (2) understanding the problem(s); and (3) managing the problem(s). The model also promotes a clear distinction between basic skills that can be developed in a relatively limited period of time and higher order skills that require considerably more time and effort to teach and learn.

The focus of this text rests on the basic skills components of the interview. For each of the three functions, therefore, the text describes a limited set of operationally defined skills that can be demonstrated and practiced in a concrete, straightforward fashion. Such operational definitions render the basic skills more teachable and easier to learn.

Expert interviewing skill, on the other hand, ultimately requires considerably more than the ability to perform a small set of operationally defined skills. Higher order skills, however, are more difficult to define and consequently more difficult to teach and learn. Some of these higher order skills and associated internal cognitive processes are described in this text. These descriptions, albeit brief, will hopefully help learners appreciate the way more complex skills can be developed upon a foundation of core competencies. Furthermore, many of these higher order skills can continue to be understood as relating to each of the three core functions of the interview. References are provided for learners interested in pursuing these more complex aspects of interviewing.

This process of differentiating basic skills from higher order skills and presenting operational definitions of the basic skills helps learners remain clear headed about what skills can be realistically attained in limited periods of time and with limited resources. It helps learners appreciate that higher order skills require considerably more effort to master. This understanding of the complexity of higher order skills can help beginners avoid the frustration many learners experience when trying to imitate truly expert interviewers who seem to accomplish so much with their patients in what appears to be such an effortless fashion. Highly skilled interviewers, in fact, have perfected a craft much as a skilled surgeon has developed his or her skill. Acknowledging that such highly tuned skills represent higher order accomplishments can help learners realize the necessity for dedicated efforts to achieve such proficiency.

This new text on the medical interview therefore seems worthwhile because it simplifies the task of learning to communicate with patients. By simplifying the task, the text strives to make the process more interesting and more relevant. Furthermore, by providing equal emphasis on each of the three separate functions of the interview, the text underscores the point that the first and third functions (i.e., the relationship and management aspects of interviewing) represent dimensions of medical care of equal importance to the second and more traditionally emphasized function of the interview (i.e., understanding the problem).

It is worth noting that the text may also be useful for audiences other than medical students. For example, the three-function model has already been used in a variety of other medical settings: internal medicine and family practice residencies, psychiatry residencies, physician assistants' programs, nursing programs, social work programs, and continuing education programs for physicians in practice.

Because of its applicability to the generic process of communication, the model has also found uses outside medicine, in the business community for programs on negotiation, and to journalism audiences for programs on interviewing. The book could be adapted for use in these other settings as well.

The medical student, however, serves as the prime focus of this text. If the book helps even a few future physicians learn better communication skills, the effort to create it will have been worthwhile. If even a few of their patients benefit, the justification for the book will be self-evident.

Steven A. Cole
Julian Bird

ACKNOWLEDGMENTS

Many patients, colleagues, mentors, and trainees have made significant contributions to this book. It is a pleasure to acknowledge our indebtedness and gratitude to them.

The original concept of the three-function model of the medical interview was developed by Julian Bird. Julian is particularly grateful to Erville Millar who, when he was notionally his trainee in the late 1970's, opened his eyes to the power of respectful and skillful clinical dialogue.

Aaron Lazare, Mack Lipkin, and Sam Putnam developed an especially robust elaboration of the original three-function concept[1] and their ideas contributed to the final product presented in this text. Ulrich Grueninger, Michael Goldstein, Penny Williamson, and Dan Duffy contributed significantly to the development of the third function of the interview (i.e., management skills).[2] Mack Lipkin, Jr., introduced us to the generative concepts and methods of learner-centered learning. We also thank him for his thoughtful and meticulous page-by-page commentary on an early version of the first edition.

We would also like to acknowledge the contributions of our colleagues in the American Academy on Patient and Physician and the UK Medical Interviewing Teaching Association (MITA). Angela Hall deserves special mention for her dedication to the development of MITA and her contributions to many ideas in this book. Rosalind Mance has been a valued colleague and contributor throughout the development of the model. She read selected portions of the manuscript and provided many useful suggestions.

We also thank Ruth Hoppe and David Steel, who were generous enough to read the manuscript and offer valuable suggestions that contributed significantly to the final product.

The following individuals all contributed chapters to the second edition of this text and have improved it immeasurably: David Steele, Kathy Cole-Kelly, Thomas Campbell, Geoff Gordon, Cecile Carson, and Dennis Novack.

Deirdre Willin, my administrative assistant, deserves special recognition and appreciation for her unfailing dedication to the completion of this project.

While all of the above individuals can rightly claim some credit for whatever strengths may be found in the text, we assume sole responsibility for the deficits.

Steven A. Cole
Julian Bird

1. Lazare A, Lipkin M Jr, Putnam SM: Three functions of the medical interview. In Lipkin M Jr, Putnam SM, Lazare A, editors: *The medical interview: clinical care, education and research,* New York, 1995, Springer-Verlag.
2. Grueninger V, Goldstein M, Duffy D: Patient education in the medical encounter: how to facilitate learning, behavior change, and coping. In Lipkin M Jr, Putnam S, Lazare A, editors: *The medical interview: clinical care, education and research,* New York, 1995, Springer-Verlag.

CONTENTS

UNIT I

THE THREE FUNCTIONS OF EFFECTIVE INTERVIEWING

CHAPTER

1 Learning to Interview by Using the Three-Function Approach

This book is about learning to communicate effectively with patients. Before anything else, a good doctor must be a good communicator. By using the interview as a clinical tool, the skilled physician strives to accomplish three broad objectives: (1) to establish and maintain an effective doctor-patient relationship; (2) to diagnose the patient's problems; and (3) to educate and motivate the patient to cooperate with treatment recommendations.

The medical interview represents the physician's core clinical tool for the diagnosis of medical conditions and the management of patients. To become proficient at the various tasks of interviewing, medical students must work hard to master basic techniques and must practice these techniques with patients. This book has been written to assist students in these efforts.

The book is structured around the three core functions of the medical interview, first described by Bird and Cohen-Cole[1] and modified by Lazare and colleagues[2]: (1) building an effective doctor-patient relationship; (2) assessing the patient's problems; and (3) managing the patient's problems. As described in this text, each of these three functions is served by a limited, pragmatic, and explicit set of operationally defined skills. *Function one* employs skills focusing on the emotional domain of the encounter. *Function two* uses data-gathering techniques. *Function three* relies primarily on adherence-management skills (education, negotiation, and motivation).

Interview training programs in medical schools have undergone significant evolution in recent years. Previously, many of these courses were focused on "history taking" as the principal goal of the communication process—that is, on only one of the three core functions of the interview. The emotional and adherence-management domains of the encounter were routinely omitted. Furthermore, even within the realm of data gathering itself, courses in medical interviewing often centered on the particular information students needed to collect by the end of the interview. These courses did not address the specific skills students needed to master in order to obtain this information efficiently; courses tended to focus on the end results or "content" of the interview, rather than on the skills needed or "process" of how to get the information.[3]

Traditional interviewing programs operated under the assumption, usually implicit, that the interpersonal skills necessary for effective interviewing either were "naturally" part of the students' repertoire or would develop through the process of accumulated medical experience. However, it has become clear that the communication skills of medical students do not improve through years of medical training. In fact, research findings and clinical experience confirm that unless students have the benefit of explicit communication skills training, their "natural" communication skills tend to deteriorate through the years of medical school and residency.[4]

Research findings, along with contemporary changes in the culture of medical education, have facilitated the emergence of medical interviewing courses that focus specifically on developing the interpersonal skills needed for efficient and effective medical interviewing. Most medical schools in the United States and Europe now provide communication skills programs of some sort. However, many of these programs lack an easily understood conceptual framework for the medical interview that would help students organize the complexities of the communication process.[5]

This text provides a tool that helps students organize the communication process. The three-function model begins with an explicit and pragmatic overview that helps students both understand the larger goals of interview training and develop the concrete skills tied to each of the three interview functions. By identifying three core functions of the interview and describing specific operationally defined skills that serve each of these core functions, the model assists students in acquiring the techniques of good interviewing that will help them throughout their medical careers.

The book is organized in such a way that each of the three core functions of the interview can be taught and learned separately. This format is artificial to some extent because, in practice, emotional and management issues overlap with the assessment process, and vice-versa. However, for the purposes of educational clarity the three functions are addressed separately.

Some programs may choose to focus on only one or two of the three functions discussed in this text. This book can easily be adapted for these approaches as well. For example, some programs may not examine management issues in medical student courses. In this case the parts of the book on the third function could be excluded. Conversely, some programs may emphasize adherence management. The book has been written so that different sections may be used separately, depending on the needs of the educational program for which it is assigned.

In Unit I, "The Three Functions of Effective Interviewing," the text begins with an elaboration of each of the three functions of the interview and a description of the specific skills useful for achieving each of the functional goals. Unit II, "Meeting the Patient," will be especially helpful for students preparing to interview patients for the first time. Within the unit, Chapter 6, "Ten Common Concerns," discusses common and anxiety-provoking questions that medical students often ask as they begin learning how to interview.

After presentation of the basic skills underlying the three core functions and discussion of common student concerns, the text systematically addresses the structural elements of the interview in Unit III, "Structure of the Interview." As described by Lipkin and associates,[6] the structural view of the interview identifies the concrete, sequential stages in which the physician actually conducts the interview. This text builds upon previous descriptions of the structure of the interview and presents a more integrated view of function and structure. This view includes "Opening" (Chapter 7), "Chief Complaint and Survey of Problems" (Chapter 8), "History of Present Illness (Problem Exploration)" (Chapter 9), "Medical History" (Chapter 10), "Family History" (Chapter 11), "Patient Profile and Social History" (Chapter 12), "Review of Systems" (Chapter 13), and "Mental Status" (Chapter 14).

In Unit IV, "Understanding the Patient's Emotional Responses," the presentation of the basic functional and structural elements is supplemented with selected advanced topics that may be useful to all interviewers, both beginners and the more experienced. Common emotional reactions to illness are reviewed in Chapter 15, "Normal Reactions." Chapter 16, "Emotional Reactions," reviews maladaptive reactions (e.g., persistent anger, anxiety, or a depressed mood).

The chapters of Unit V, "Managing Communication Challenges," suggest pragmatic clinical approaches to each of eight challenging interview situations: "Sexual Issues in the Interview" (Chapter 17), "Interviewing Elderly Patients" (Chapter 18), "Overcoming Cultural and Language Barriers" (Chapter 19), "Family Interviewing" (Chapter 20), "Troubling Personality Styles and Somatization" (Chapter 21), "Nonadherence, Lifestyle Change, and Stress" (Chapter 22), "Psychosis, Delirium, and Dementia" (Chapter 23), and "Breaking Bad News" (Chapter 24).

The four chapters of Unit VI, "Higher-Order Skills," address the higher-order skills that physicians must master to develop the high level of proficiency required for the effective practice of clinical medicine: "Nonverbal Communication" (Chapter 25), "Use of the Self in Medical Care" (Chapter 26), "Using Psychologic Principles in the Medical Interview" (Chapter 27), and "Integrating Structure and Function" (Chapter 28). Appendix One focuses on the learning process itself. The appendix discusses several different educational approaches and the use of different techniques for those who wish to learn better interviewing skills. Finally, Appendix Two contains a table displaying all the basic skills of the model.

The text can be useful not only for medical students, but also for a variety of other audiences. The three-function model of the interview has already been used successfully in several other educational settings in medicine: internal medicine and family practice residencies, psychiatry residencies, physician assistants' programs, nursing programs, social work and psychology programs, and continuing education programs for physicians in practice. In addition, the model has found applications outside medicine, in the business community for programs on negotiation, and in journalism and correctional (police) work for programs on interviewing. This book can be adapted for use in these other settings as well.

REFERENCES

1. Bird J, Cohen-Cole SA: The three function model of the medical interview: an educational device. In Hale M, editor: *Models of consultation-liaison psychiatry,* Basel, Switzerland, 1990, Karger, pp 65-88.
2. Lazare A, Putnam SM, Lipkin M Jr: Three functions of the medical interview. In Lipkin M Jr, Putnam SM, Lazare A, editors: *The medical interview: clinical care, education, and research,* New York, 1995, Springer, pp 3-19.
3. Stoeckle JD, Billings JA: A history of history-taking: the medical interview, *J Gen Intern Med* 2 (2):119-127, 1987.
4. Carroll JG, Lipkin M Jr, Nachtigall L, et al: A developmental awareness for teaching doctor/patient communication skills. In Lipkin M Jr, Putnam SM, Lazare A, editors: *The medical interview: clinical care, education, and research,* New York, 1995, Springer, pp 388-396.
5. Novack DH, Volk G, Drossman DA, et al: Medical interviewing and interpersonal skills teaching in U.S. medical schools: progress, problems, and promise, *JAMA* 270:1319-1320, 1993.
6. Lipkin M: The medical interview and related skills. In Branch WT, editor: *The office practice of medicine,* ed 3, Philadelphia, 1994, WB Saunders.

CHAPTER

2 Why Three Functions?

The three-function model of the medical interview was created to help students master the basic skills of communicating with patients. The three functions described in the model do not encompass every aspect of medical interviewing, only the core essentials that students should develop before they face the challenges of developing higher-order skills.

The three functions of the interview described in this text include (1) building the relationship; (2) assessing the patient's problems; and (3) managing the patient's problems. Each of these functions is associated with a specific set of operationally defined interviewing behaviors that can help the student achieve the objectives related to the function. The book describes each of the interviewing behaviors in detail and demonstrates how these skills can be used in the process of patient interviewing. This chapter focuses on the underlying reasons that each of the three core functions is critically important for the efficient and effective practice of medicine.

THE FIRST FUNCTION: BUILDING THE RELATIONSHIP

The first function of the interview addresses the physician's primary task: to build and maintain an effective doctor-patient relationship.[1,2] An effective partnership serves as the foundation for the rest of the interview, as well as for the entire process of medical care. Conversely, a troubled doctor-patient relationship leads to inefficient assessment and problematic management. The experienced physician uses relationship-building skills from the first moment of the interview and throughout the assessment and management process.

In general, physicians build the relationship by attending to the *emotional* domain of the patient's problems. The experience of illness arouses intense emotions for patients and their families. Pain, discomfort, disability, and death (or the threat of death) inevitably raise numerous and sometimes complex emotional reactions. Individuals and families facing illness situations frequently experience anxiety about the unknown, sadness or depression about losses or potential losses, and anger about the impact of illness on overall life adjustment.

All patients must deal with the emotional domain of illness. The child with juvenile-onset diabetes must cope with the lifelong burden of chronic illness and the impact of this illness on peer relationships, school adjustment, and family life. The young mother with multiple sclerosis faces a future of uncertain disability with frightening implications for her ability to care for her children in the way she would like. The middle-aged executive with coronary artery disease has to deal with a life-threatening illness that may affect income, career opportunities, and overall quality of life. Furthermore, the management of coronary artery disease usually entails the additional burden of major life-style changes (e.g., smoking behavior, diet, and exercise). The terminal cancer patient and the patient's family must find a way to deal with the inevitability of death and the associated emotional turmoil. Each of these emotionally charged illness situations leads to differing types of reactions in different individuals.

The manner in which the physician responds to the common emotions associated with illness will, to a large extent, determine the quality of overall doctor-patient rapport, affect patient adherence and adaptation, and influence the physiologic course and outcome of the illness. The empirical literature upon which these assertions rest is extensive. A few of the numerous supporting studies are described. Mumford and associates,[3] for example, reviewed 34 controlled studies of emotionally supportive or educational interventions after surgery or myocardial infarctions. Patients in the experimental groups suffered fewer physical and emotional complications of illness and were discharged from hospitals an average of 2 days earlier than were patients in the control groups. Other studies indicate that patients who are more satisfied with their physicians are more likely to adhere to treatment recommendations and that physicians who are more skilled in the emotional domain of patient interaction are likely to have more satisfied patients.[4] Health care providers who have been trained in interviewing skills have been shown to be better able to detect and manage emotional distress in their patients.[5] Similarly, patient centeredness on the part of the physician, partnership, and participatory decision making between the physician and the patient have been shown to lead to improved physical outcome in hypertension, diabetes, and arthritis.[6]

In general, the research documenting the relevance of the physician-patient relationship to the outcome of illness emanates from a theoretical perspective called the "biopsychosocial model of illness."[7] This view of illness asserts that psychologic and social variables play a key role in the development, course, and outcome of all illnesses. Persuasive scientific evidence supports this model of illness: (1) stressful life events are associated in numerous studies with the subsequent development of physical illnesses; (2) low social support has been associated in prospective studies with subsequent death, even after controlling for other health-related variables such as previous health status, smoking, visits to the doctor, and social class; (3) the combination of low social support and high stress after an initial heart attack is associated with a threefold risk of a subsequent heart attack; (4) group therapy has been shown to be associated with increased longevity in randomized, controlled, prospective studies of patients with breast cancer and malignant melanoma; and (5) major depression, as well as other psychosocial stressors, has been associated with suppression of the immune system.[8] Other reviews of these data are now available.[9]

A basic tenet of the biopsychosocial model of illness is that optimal patient care will be delivered by physicians who are aware of the psychosocial dimensions of illness and skilled in the assessment and management of these variables. The three-function model of the medical interview has been uniquely designed to serve as the vehicle for applying the biopsychosocial model in actual clinical practice. In particular, the elaboration of the first function explicitly addresses the need for physicians to attend to the psychologic, emotional, and relational aspects of their communication with their patients. Because the emotional domain of medical practice plays such a key role in the determination of medical outcome, students will become better doctors by focusing their attention on learning the explicit communication skills that improve their competencies in this area.

To be sure, most students and physicians already possess intuitive abilities to respond to patients' emotions. In many situations, helping a patient who is anxious or sad may simply require the use of "natural" empathic skills. As Peabody pointed out in a classic article:

> One of the essential qualities of the physician is interest in humanity, for the secret of the care of the patient is caring for the patient.[10]

On the other hand, numerous studies, clinical observations, and physicians' responses to surveys indicate that this intuitive ability may not be sufficient. The intensity of busy practices and the wide variety of patients' emotional responses understandably demand more knowledge and skill in the emotional domain of doctor-patient relationship building than many practitioners naturally possess without added training. For example, while approximately 20% of medical patients suffer from significant psychiatric disorders (primarily anxiety, depression, and substance abuse), studies indicate that at least half of these disorders are not recognized by physicians.[11] Medical school experiences that do not explicitly address the recognition and management of the emotional and psychiatric aspects of general medical illness may therefore not prepare students adequately for their future practice of medicine.

The first function of the three-function model of the medical interview focuses on the emotional domain of clinical practice. Five skills are described that can be demonstrated and practiced by students to help them master some basic approaches to this difficult aspect of medical interviewing. Although there are certainly numerous other ways to effectively respond to patients' emotions, students who master the five basic interventions described in this book will be better able to integrate these responses with their own natural inclinations and abilities. Furthermore, recent studies indicate that physicians who are better able to respond to patients' emotional distress report higher satisfaction of their own.[12]

Students interested in learning more sophisticated strategies for helping patients cope with emotions (including supportive, insight-oriented, cognitive, or behavioral strategies) can appropriately build these higher-order skills upon the foundation of the basic skills described in this text.[13]

THE SECOND FUNCTION: ASSESSING THE PATIENT'S PROBLEMS

The second function of the interview concerns the need to obtain information to assess the patient's problems. Experts rate the interview as more important than either the physical examination or the laboratory investigation for making accurate diagnoses. Perhaps three fourths of all diagnoses can still be made based on the history alone, despite the technologic innovations of modern medicine.[14] The skillful physician uses data-gathering skills to assess the patient's problems and arrive at diagnostic formulations.

Collecting accurate information in a time-efficient manner is also recognized as a universal goal for physicians. Occasionally, these two goals (accuracy and brevity) may be in opposition. For example, in an effort to be efficient, physicians may rush their patients and miss important information. In fact, one recent study demonstrated this problem clearly. Beckman and Frankel[15] tape-recorded interviews between internists and their patients and found that in 69% of interviews, physicians interrupted their patients within the first 18 seconds of the encounter. Of even greater concern, these interruptions led to the decreased accuracy of the physicians' understanding of the patients' problems and to incomplete collection of data. In 77% of the interviews the patients' reasons for coming to the physicians were not fully elicited.[15]

The seminal and widely cited study conducted by Beckman and Frankel was published in 1984. Since that time, many medical schools have developed interviewing skills programs to address these problems, and the medical literature continues to emphasize that practicing physicians attend to these problems in their own practices. The study was recently repeated in another city, with nearly identical results. Unfortunately, these findings indicate the continued existence of the problems and the need for attention to training in communication skills for increased medical effectiveness and efficiency.[16]

The goal of the second function of the interview is the collection of accurate, sufficient, and relevant data from the patient in as efficient a manner as possible. A few specific doctor behaviors or skills can contribute to the achievement of this goal. These skills are reviewed in the next chapter.

THE THIRD FUNCTION: MANAGING THE PATIENT'S PROBLEMS

Physicians rely on the third function of the interview to educate patients and to motivate them to adhere to treatment recommendations. Successful management requires the use of educational, negotiation, and motivational skills in the interview. Because the third function addresses all three of these separate but related skills, it is the most complex of the three functions of the interview.

Patients do not understand their doctors very well. For example, when patients are asked to discuss their illness and its treatment (even immediately after leaving their physicians' offices), they can correctly identify only about 50% of critical information.[17] Other research shows that about 50% of patients do not know what medicines they are supposed to take. It is clear that many patients are poorly informed about their illness and treatment. Some of this lack of information may be attributable to inadequate patient education by physicians. It seems reasonable that physicians who learn to communicate information better will have patients who understand more about their illness and who will be more likely to adhere to treatment recommendations.[18]

Patient nonadherence is also a major problem in current medical practice. Hundreds of studies indicate that between 22% and 72% of patients do not follow their doctor's recommendations. The percentage of nonadherent patients varies according to illness category (e.g., 23% nonadherence in medications for acute illness vs. 45% for illness prevention) and outcome measured (e.g., 54% nonadherence to appointments for prevention and 72% nonadherence to diets). It is worth noting, however, that these numbers do not vary according to the educational level or socioeconomic status of the patient.[19]

Many physicians spend a great deal of time trying to educate or motivate patients, but few practitioners have received any training in strategies to do this efficiently or effectively. There is good evidence that such training can improve physician skill, patient knowledge, patient satisfaction, and, ultimately, patient adherence and physical outcome.[20]

Recent evidence has underscored the relationship between certain life-style behaviors (e.g., overeating, alcohol consumption, tobacco use, and a lack of exercise) and negative health consequences. Physicians are becoming increasingly involved with attempts to influence patients' high-risk health behaviors. To achieve effectiveness in such areas, physicians can benefit from training in the empirically validated strategies that help patients change these behaviors.[18]

This text raises communication strategies regarding education, negotiation, and motivation to a level of importance equal to that of assessment and relationship building. To be sure, the ultimate impact of a physician's assessment or rapport-building skills cn patient care may be entirely undermined by his or her inability to achieve patient adherence to treatment recommendations. Therefore a concrete and pragmatic set of educational, negotiation, and motivational strategies has been recommended for all medical student education. Students interested in developing higher-order skills in this area will be directed to other sources for future learning.

REFERENCES

1. Tresolini CP, The Pew-Fetzer Task Force: *Health professions education and relationship centered care,* San Francisco, 1994, Pew Health Professions Commission.
2. Suchman AL, Hinton-Walker P, Botelho RJ, editors: *Partnerships in healthcare: transforming relational process,* Rochester, NY, 1998, University of Rochester Press.
3. Mumford E, Schlesinger HJ, Glass GV: The effects of psychological intervention on recovery from surgery and heart attacks: an analysis of the literature, *Am J Public Health* 72:141-151, 1982.
4. Roter D, Hall J: *Doctors talking to patients/patients talking to doctors,* Westport, Conn, 1992, Auburn House.
5. Roter DL, Hall JA, Kern DE, et al: Improving physicians' interviewing skills and reducing patients' emotional distress, *Arch Intern Med* 155:1877-1884, 1995.
6. Stewart MA: Effective physician-patient communication and health outcomes: a review, *Can Med Assoc J* 152:1423-1433, 1995.
7. Engel GL: The need for a new medical model: a challenge for biomedicine, *Science* 196:129-136, 1974.
8. Cole S, Saravay S, Levinson R: The biopsychosocial model of illness. In Stoudemire A, editor: *Human behavior: an introduction to human behavior,* ed 3, Philadelphia, 1998, JB Lippincott, pp 36-84.
9. Walker E, Katon W: Psychological factors affecting physical conditions and responses to stress. In Stoudemire A, editor: *Clinical psychiatry for medical students,* Philadelphia, 1990, JB Lippincott.
10. Peabody FW: The care of the patient, *JAMA* 88:877-882, 1927.
11. Lin EH, Simon GE, Katon WJ, et al: Can enhanced acute-phase treatment of depression improve long-term outcomes? a report of randomized trials in primary care, *Am J Psychiatr* 156(4):643-645, 1999.

12. Suchman AL, Roter DL, Greene MG, et al: Physician satisfaction with primary care office visits, *Med Care* 31:1083-1092, 1993.
13. Novack D: Therapeutic aspects of the clinical encounter, *J Gen Intern Med* 2:346-354, 1987.
14. Peterson MC, Holbrook JH, Voon Hales MD: Contributions of the history, physical examination, and laboratory investigation in making medical diagnoses, *West J Med* 15:163-165, 1992.
15. Beckman HB, Frankel RM: The effect of physician behavior on the collection of data, *Ann Intern Med* 101:692-696, 1984.
16. Marvel K, Epstein R, Flowers K, et al: Soliciting the patients' agenda: have we improved? *JAMA* 281(3):283-287, 1999.
17. Stewart M: Patient recall and comprehension after the medical visit. In Lipkin M Jr, Putnam SM, Lazare A, editors: *The medical interview: clinical care, education, and research,* New York, 1995, Springer, pp 525-529.
18. Grueninger U, Duffy DF, Goldstein M: Patient education in the medical encounter: how to facilitate learning, behavior change, and coping. In Lipkin M Jr, Putnam SM, Lazare A, editors: *The medical interview: clinical care, education, and research,* New York, 1995, Springer, pp 122-123.
19. Dye N, DiMatteo MR: Enhancing cooperation with the medical regimen. In Lipkin M Jr, Putnam SM, Lazare A, editors: *The medical interview: clinical care, education, and research,* New York, 1995, Springer, pp 134-136.
20. Stewart MA: Effective physician-patient communication and health outcomes: a review, *Can Med Assoc J* 159:1423-1433, 1995.

CHAPTER

3 Function One: Building the Relationship

The physician-patient relationship stands as the cornerstone of clinical medicine. The first function of the interview, "Building the Relationship," uses a set of emotional response skills, which are among the most important communication skills the physician can develop.

Patients expect their doctors to be knowledgeable and technically competent. But they also want and need their doctors to be reassuring, supportive, and emotionally available. The physician with good relationship skills will have patients who are more satisfied and who will be more likely to adhere to treatment recommendations.[1] Furthermore, the physician with good relationship skills will cope with emotionally troubling situations better and will, in general, find the clinical practice of medicine more enjoyable. Such a physician will be able to give more to patients emotionally and will, in turn, get more satisfying responses from them.

This chapter describes a group of basic relationship skills that help build doctor-patient rapport: (1) nonverbal skills; (2) empathy; (3) partnership; (4) support; and (5) respect. Once learned, these skills can be integrated into the student's or physician's natural response set and can then provide the foundation for interested learners to master higher-order skills for continued relationship building or for helping patients cope better with emotional distress.

NONVERBAL SKILLS

The nonverbal behavior of the physician may be the most important single determinant of the quality of the overall doctor-patient relationship. Appropriate body posture, body movements, facial expression, voice tone and rate of speech, touch, and the space between doctor and patient can convey an attitude of concern and warmth far beyond any words that may be uttered.[2] The level of the doctor's interest in the patient is communicated nonverbally.

Physicians should strive for consistency between their verbal and nonverbal behavior. For example, if there is a disjunction between the doctor's verbal statements of concern and his or her nonverbal behavior (which may, for example, indicate boredom or contempt), the nonverbal message will usually prevail in the patient's mind.[3]

An emerging body of research supports contentions about the importance of doctors' nonverbal behavior. Doctors who establish appropriate eye contact are more likely to detect emotional distress in their patients. Doctors who perform better on tests of nonverbal sensitivity have patients who are more satisfied. Doctors who lean forward and have a forward head lean and open body posture also have more satisfied patients.[4]

In addition, the nonverbal behavior of the patients is a key to their emotional lives. Most patients express their emotional states through facial expressions, body posture, movement, tone of voice, inflection, and physical manifestations of autonomic nervous system reactivity (e.g., sweaty palms or a flushed face). Skilled physicians will always be interested in understanding their patients' emotional states and will therefore always look for these signs and consider their importance at every stage of the communication process.

In general, physicians should establish and keep comfortable eye contact with their patients throughout the interview. This is essential to listening actively and effectively and to observing new emotional cues as they arise. As with all rules, there are exceptions; angry, suspicious, or paranoid patients may perceive steady, unrelieved eye contact as provocative.

Thoughtful attention to the use of space also facilitates rapport. Vertical space between the doctor and patient (e.g., not standing while the patient sits) should be minimized and horizontal space (e.g., not too close or too far) should be carefully planned. Chapter 25 on nonverbal communication discusses all of these issues in more depth.

EMPATHY

"Empathy" is a term indicating one person's appreciation, understanding, and acceptance of someone else's emotional situation. The communication of this understanding is one of the most helpful, meaningful, and comforting interventions one person can have with another. A parent soothes an upset child by letting the child know that the distress is understood, appreciated, and accepted. Friends and lovers do the same. Similarly, a physician can best build rapport and respond to patients' emotions by communicating empathy.[5]

The communication of an empathic understanding of a patient's predicament is clearly the most important relationship-building skill the physician can possess. There are many different ways to communicate empathy effectively. The challenge of learning empathic skills lies in developing the ability to master basic interventions and to integrate these into a natural interpersonal style that feels genuine to the interviewer and, as such, is likely to be perceived as genuine by the patient.

Nonverbal behaviors can sometimes communicate empathy more effectively than can concrete statements. A sympathetic look, an attentive silence, and a hand on the shoulder can all accomplish a great deal toward letting the patient know the doctor is emotionally in tune with the patient's distress.

Many medical students and, indeed, practicing physicians believe that empathic understanding and the ability to communicate empathetically are basic human traits and that these skills cannot be taught. However, research evidence indicates the contrary. Medical students demonstrate significant deficiencies in empathic communication and do not improve throughout their training.[6] Education can improve empathic abilities; randomized, controlled trials indicate that students and practicing physicians who have participated in targeted training programs or communication workshops have improved these skills, with consequent improvement in patient outcome.[7-10]

Most physicians already possess considerable empathic abilities, but the challenges of medical practice often require the development of additional skills. Once learned, these skills can be integrated into the clinician's natural repertoire.

This chapter describes two operational components of empathic communication, *reflection* and *legitimation,* that can be used to facilitate the physician's response to patients' emotional distress. "Reflection" refers to the physician's describing the emotion experienced by the patient, and "legitimation" refers to the physician's confirming that the emotion is understood and accepted.

Reflection

Reflection is a straightforward concept drawn from rogerian psychology. It refers to a physician's statement of an observed feeling or emotion in the patient.[11] For example, when the physician notices that a patient begins to look sad when discussing the illness of a parent, the physician can "reflect" this feeling by saying something like the following:

> **Physician:** You look a bit sad right now.
> *or*
> I can see this is upsetting to you.
> *or*
> This is hard to talk about.

This type of reflective comment usually helps the physician communicate empathic concern for the patient's emotional situation. In practical terms, such physician comments usually give the patient permission to talk more about the feelings that are being experienced.

The specific words are much less important than the fact that the physician has interrupted the factual exchange of information to notice and respond to the patient's emotional state. This is a critically important event in the building of a relationship with the patient and demonstrates to the patient that the doctor is concerned about the patient as a person and about his or her emotional experiences.

An example of a reflective comment might occur just after a physician notices that a patient looks sad or teary eyed. The physician might say the following in a supportive tone of voice:

Physician: I can see that you seem a bit upset right now.

Sometimes physicians are reluctant to use reflective comments to encourage the patient to express feelings more deeply. Doctors may feel that this will open a Pandora's box of emotions or that empathic comments will push patients to express feelings that they might otherwise wish to keep private. To the contrary, it is helpful and supportive to allow patients at least some opportunity for the ventilation of feelings that are near the surface of awareness. Such interventions help develop rapport and also contribute to the overall efficiency of the interview. Although some physicians may believe that attention to the emotional domain of patient care increases interview time, research indicates that empathic communication improves numerous outcomes of importance (e.g., patient satisfaction, disclosure of information, and decreased emotional distress) *without increasing overall interview time.*[12,13]

In general, initial reflective comments should be presented in a manner that is the least threatening to a patient and in terms the patient is likely to accept. Lazare[14] has correctly pointed out that the premature use of terminology indicating levels of emotion deeper than the patient is ready to acknowledge may interfere with rapport or, even worse, lead to the patient's experiencing guilt or shame. For example, the angry patient should be told, "You seem a bit irritated," rather than, "You seem very angry." Similarly, a depressed patient should be told initially, "I can tell you're down," rather than, "You seem to be in despair."

If patients at this point indicate that they do not wish to discuss their emotional reactions, physicians should of course respect these desires. However, it is important that the physician not confuse his or her own desire to avoid emotional issues with the inference that it is the patient who wishes to avoid these topics. If the physician does not acknowledge the patient's manifest feelings, the patient will feel unconfirmed and less understood. Such feelings undermine doctor-patient rapport and actually interfere with the collection of data. In addition to the usefulness of emotional ventilation for the task of data collection, patients who feel understood by their physicians are generally more satisfied and feel better.[15]

This leads to better doctor-patient rapport, a more satisfying relationship for physicians, better detection of psychiatric illness,[13] better physical outcome,[16] and fewer lawsuits.[17,18]

The following suggestion stands as one of the cardinal rules of good interviewing:

Respond to a patient's feeling as soon as it appears.

The physician who avoids acknowledging a patient's feeling may give the patient the message that he or she is afraid of the feeling or, worse, uninterested.

It is useful for physicians to remember that reflective comments can be used several times as a patient discusses and experiences feelings. One reflective comment is often insufficient. In fact, as a patient ventilates emotional reactions, the specific feeling expressed may change in quality and degree. For example, a patient who seems sad at first may eventually express frustration, or vice-versa. If the physician listens carefully, the initial feeling can be acknowledged and subsequent ones reflected as they emerge.

Attention to patients' feelings usually does not require excessive time. If the emotional issues clearly become too complex to address in the interview time available, the physician can acknowledge the significance of the feelings and make arrangements to deal with the emotional issues at a later, but acceptable, date. Alternatively, a suitable alternate approach (e.g., a psychiatric, psychologic, or social work referral) could be arranged.

Legitimation

Legitimation, or validation, is closely related to reflection but indicates an intervention that specifically communicates acceptance of and respect for the patient's emotional experience. After a physician has carefully listened to the patient's discussion of an emotional reaction, the physician should let the patient know that the feelings are understandable and make sense to the physician. The following are examples of validating comments:

Physician: I can certainly understand why you'd be upset under the circumstances.

or

Anyone would find this very difficult.

or

Your reactions are perfectly normal.

or

This would be anxiety provoking for anyone.

or

I can understand why you're so angry.

With respect to validating the feelings of someone who is angry, it is important to realize that the physician does not have to agree with the reasons for the anger. The important point to remember is that it is important to try to understand this anger from the patient's point of view. Once the physician has understood the anger, this understanding can be communicated to the patient. This is sometimes difficult to do if the physician disagrees with or feels irritated or threatened by an angry patient. Nevertheless, reflective and validating comments can play the same helpful role with angry patients as they do with sad or anxious patients. For example, if the patient is angry because he or she has been waiting too long (an occurrence that happens all too frequently), the physician may appropriately say:

Physician: I can see that you are frustrated because you've been waiting so long. I understand why you are angry. I am truly sorry, but there really wasn't anything I could do about it.

In a more threatening situation, when the physician feels accused of making a mistake but does not think a mistake has been made, the following type of comment can be helpful:

Physician: I can understand that you feel a mistake has been made. I also understand that this has made you very angry. I have to let you know that I do not agree with you that a mistake has been made. However, I can understand why you feel so angry.

These principles are discussed at greater length in Chapters 15 and 16 on strategies for interviewing patients with troubling emotions or behaviors.

PERSONAL SUPPORT

Statements of personal support can enhance rapport. The physician should make explicit efforts to let the patient know that he or she is there, personally, for the patient and wants to help. Of course, this must be an honest statement, or it will not be effective. Statements like the following indicate personal support:

Physician: I want to help in any way I can.
or
Let me know what I can do to help.

These types of statements of direct personal support encourage the patient to feel that the physician wants to help, leading to improved rapport and solidification of the doctor-patient relationship.

PARTNERSHIP

Patients are more satisfied with physicians and are more likely to adhere to treatment recommendations when they feel a sense of partnership with their physicians.[19] Increasing the participation of patients in their own treatment improves their coping skills and increases the likelihood of good outcome from illness processes.[20] When physicians are interested and willing to promote this type of partnership, they can make such statements as these:

> **Physician:** Let's work together in developing a treatment plan once I have reviewed some of the options with you.
>
> *or*
>
> After we've talked some more about your problems, perhaps together we can work out some solutions that may help.

RESPECT

The physician's respect for patients and their problems is implied by attentive listening, nonverbal signals, eye contact, and genuine concern. However, explicit, respectful comments also help build rapport, improve the relationship, and help the patient cope with difficult situations.

For the purposes of this text, an intervention communicating respect refers to a specific endorsement for a specific patient behavior. Statements of respect, which validate patient behaviors, will, in general, tend to reinforce the behavior and make it more likely to happen again. Frequent demonstrations of respect will foster a positive relationship and promote the patients' capacity for coping.

Physicians can usually find something to praise in all their patients. Almost everyone does something well. This holds true even for patients with troubling or difficult behaviors (see Chapter 21). Doctors can help their patients by focusing on one or more of their patients' successful coping skills. This can also improve patient satisfaction and adherence. The following are examples of respectful statements:

> **Physician:** I'm impressed by how well you're coping.
>
> *or*
>
> You're doing a good job handling the uncertainty.
>
> *or*
>
> Despite your feeling so bad, you're still able to carry on at home and at work. That is quite an accomplishment.

Like all the other interventions discussed above, statements of respect must be honest, or they will be more destructive than helpful. When these sentiments reflect true feelings of the physician, however, they are powerful facilitators of improved communication and rapport between doctors and patients.

REFERENCES

1. Hall JA: Affective and nonverbal aspects of the medical visit. In Lipkin M Jr, Putnam SM, Lazare A, editors: *The medical interview: clinical care, education, and research,* New York, 1995, Springer, pp 495-503.
2. Harrigan JA, Oxman TE, Rosenthal R: Rapport expressed through nonverbal behavior, *J Nonverbal Behav* 9:95-110, 1985.
3. McCroskey JC, Larson CE, Knapp ML: *An introduction to interpersonal communication,* Englewood Cliffs, NJ, 1971, Prentice-Hall.
4. Hall JA, Harrigan JA, Rosenthal R: Non-verbal behavior in clinician-patient interaction, *Appl Prevent Psychol* 4:21-35, 1995.
5. Bellet PS, Maloney MJ: The importance of empathy as an interviewing skill in medicine, *JAMA* 266:1831-1832, 1991.
6. Suchman AL, Markakis K, Beckman H, et al: A model of empathic communication in the medical interview, *JAMA* 277:678-682, 1997.
7. Roter DL, Hall JA, Kern DE, et al: Improving physicians' interviewing skills and reducing patients' emotional distress, *Arch Intern Med* 155:1877-1884, 1995.
8. Platt FW, Keller VF: Empathic communication: a teachable and learnable skill, *J Gen Intern Med* 9:222-226, 1994.
9. Spiro H: What is empathy and can it be taught? *Ann Intern Med* 16:843-846, 1992.
10. Gerrity M, Cole S, Dietrich A, et al: Improving the recognition and management of depression: is there a role for physician education? *J Fam Pract* 48: 949-957, 1999.
11. Carkhuff RR: *Helping and human relations,* vols 1 and 2, New York, 1969, Holt, Rinehart, and Winston, pp 1-298, 1-343.
12. Levinson W, Roter D: Physicians' psychosocial beliefs correlate with their patient communication skills, *J Gen Intern Med* 10:375-379, 1995.
13. Roter DL, Hall JA, Kern DE, et al: Improving physicians' interviewing skills and reducing patients' emotional distress, *Arch Intern Med* 155:1877-1884, 1995.
14. Lazare A: Shame and humiliation in the medical encounter, *Arch Intern Med* 147:1653-1658, 1987.
15. Elstein A: Psychological research on diagnostic reasoning. In Lipkin M Jr, Putnam SM, Lazare A, editors: *The medical interview: clinical care, education, and research,* New York, 1995, Springer, pp 504-510.
16. Kaplan SH, Greenfield S, Ware JS: Impact of the doctor-patient relationship on the outcome of chronic disease. In Stewart M, Roter D, editors: *Communicating with medical patients,* London, 1989, Sage Publications, pp 228-245.
17. Cole S: Reducing malpractice risk through more effective communication, *Am J Managed Care* 3:485-489, 1997.
18. Levinson W, Roter DL, Mullooly JP, et al: The relationship with malpractice claims among primary care physicians and surgeons, *JAMA* 277:553-559, 1997.

19. Dye N, DiMatteo MR: Enhancing cooperation with the medial regimen. In Lipkin M Jr, Putnam SM, Lazare A, editors: *The medical interview: clinical care, education, and research,* New York, 1995, Springer, pp 134-146.
20. Grueninger U, Duffy DF, Goldstein M: Patient education in the medical encounter: how to facilitate learning, behavior change, and coping. In Lipkin M Jr, Putnam SM, Lazare A, editors: *The medical interview: clinical care, education, and research,* New York, 1995, Springer, pp 122-133.

CHAPTER

4 Function Two: Assessing the Patient's Problems

Listen to the patient, he is telling you the diagnosis.

Sir William Osler

After the doctor-patient relationship has been established, the second core function of the interview addresses the physician's need to assess the patient's problems. This requires the ability to listen well and to elicit information from the patient. The importance of skillful data collection is underscored by the widely accepted understanding that the medical history contributes 60% to 80% of the information needed for accurate diagnoses.[2]

This chapter describes a range of skills that have been shown to enhance the ability of physicians to collect information from patients accurately and efficiently. In the actual practice of medicine, experienced physicians develop and test diagnostic hypotheses as part of the process of collecting information from patients.[3] Thus physicians' awareness of illness patterns guides their interviewing strategies. Even without this knowledge base and experience, however, medical students can significantly improve their data-gathering efficiency by focusing on the basic skills described in this chapter.[4]

NONVERBAL LISTENING BEHAVIOR

The doctor's nonverbal behavior has a powerful effect on the flow of information. Appropriate nonverbal signals are essential. Patients will usually continue speaking when they feel their physician is listening. Physicians who look at their patients and maintain an attentive and interested body posture will be more likely to instill confidence and trust than doctors who retreat behind a desk, slouch in a chair, drink coffee while talking, or try to read or write in the chart while also trying to listen.

Appropriate eye contact is an essential first ingredient for collecting information from patients. In general, to listen well to a patient and to watch for emotional cues, the physician must look directly at the patient. In addition, an attentive body posture is crucial; for example, an open body position, a forward lean of the head, and a forward lean of the body all indicate receptivity to the patient and a willingness to listen. Although these recommendations may seem straightforward and obvious, they are commonly neglected in actual practice, and the student who begins a career with attention to such nonverbal cues will learn good habits for a lifetime of practice.

QUESTIONING STYLE: OPEN-ENDED QUESTIONS AND THE OPEN-TO-CLOSED CONE

Open-ended questions are particularly crucial in the opening of the interview and for opening up new topics as they arise. A considerable body of literature supports the use of open-ended questioning as the most efficient and effective vehicle to gain an accurate and complete understanding of patients' problems.[5-8]

An open-ended (or nondirective) question invites the patient to use his or her own judgment in deciding what topics and problems to emphasize. Open-ended questions require patients to generate responses other than a simple yes or no. The following are examples of open-ended questions:

Physician: What problems brought you to the hospital?
or
How can I be of help to you today?

In contrast, closed questions can be answered with one word. The following are examples of closed questions:

Physician: Does your head hurt?
or
Are you short of breath?
or
Is the chest pain sharp?

Open-ended questions invite patients to describe their problems by using their own vocabulary and their personal experience of the symptoms. Such questioning will much more likely lead to the physician's gaining an accurate understanding of patients' personal experience of illness. In contrast, premature reliance on closed questioning can lead to inaccurate or incomplete understanding.

Open-ended questioning is particularly useful because it allows a patient to inform the doctor about the problem as the patient sees it. Such questioning indicates the willingness of the doctor to listen to the patient's story. By using open-ended questioning in the beginning of the interview, the physician can learn more about the patient's perception of the problem, the major concerns about the problem, the context of the problem, and perhaps the deeper meaning of the problem to the patient. Such information will be invaluable to the physician in developing diagnostic hypotheses and management strategies.

After an initial nondirective phase, during which the physician has allowed the patient to speak freely about the problems as the patient sees them, the doctor must ask progressively more focused questions to explore specific diagnostic hypotheses. This subsequent graduated narrowing of focus (after initial open-ended inquiries) has been called an "open-to-closed cone."[9]

Consider the example of a young man with headaches. After the patient indicates that headaches are his major problem, the physician may choose one of two very different approaches: the physician may explore the problem of the headaches in an open-ended manner or, alternatively, rely on closed-ended inquiries to learn more about specific physical symptoms. The closed-ended approach might include many detailed questions about the location of the pain, intensity, timing, quality, and so on. These are important questions and need to be asked but should be reserved until after the initial, more open-ended exploration has been completed.

An example of a closed-ended sequence might be the following:

Physician: What can I do for you today?
Patient: I've been having terrible headaches.
Physician: I'm sorry. Where is the pain?
Patient: The pain is all over.
Physician: Is the pain sharp or dull?
Patient: Dull.

In this sequence of closed-ended questioning, the physician has not learned as much as might be gained from more open-ended inquiries.

In contrast, a more open-ended inquiry is usually more efficient in leading to diagnostic hypotheses:

Physician: Can you tell me some more about the headaches?
Patient: Well, they come on slowly and get worse and worse over several days. They seem to come only in the hay fever season when my allergies get worse.

Experienced physicians develop diagnostic hypotheses from the first moments of meeting a patient.[3] These hypotheses are formulated by fitting patterns of the patient's complaints and physical signs into entities of known illness categories. By allowing the patient the opportunity to describe his or her own complaints in a nondirected way, the skilled physician can more efficiently develop diagnostic hypotheses and recognize patterns that are relevant for the particular patient's problems.

In the open-ended example given above, the patient's description of the symptoms allows the physician to narrow the set of diagnostic possibilities considerably, even within the first few moments of the interview. The open-ended inquiry has suggested an allergic etiology for the headaches rather than numerous others. In contrast, the closed-ended inquiry was significantly less efficient. Although beginning medical students will not be able to recognize the hundreds of patterns that will soon become commonplace to them, it will be particularly useful for students to learn good habits of open-ended questioning early in their careers.

In addition, open-ended questioning usually provides the physician the opportunity to learn about the important environmental precipitants or stress factors that may influence the development of symptoms. For example, this same complaint of headaches might lead to the following:

Physician: Can you tell me some more about your headaches?
Patient: Well, they only started about three weeks ago and seem to come on when I'm in the library late at night studying for exams.

This information can help the physician understand the environmental context of the symptoms, which will help in the formulation of diagnostic hypotheses and treatment strategies. The context of late-night headaches may suggest problems with fatigue or excessive caffeine intake. In addition, the mentioning of exams suggests the possibility of stressful life situations that may be related to the headaches.

LET THE PATIENT COMPLETE THE OPENING STATEMENT.

Beckman and Frankel's research report in 1984,[11] replicated in 1999,[12] documents the importance of allowing the patient to complete his or her opening statement. While most medical interviews do begin with open-ended questioning, in at least 75% of interviews, physicians typically interrupt their patients before they get the chance to complete their initial thoughts, generally within the first 20 seconds of the interview! Most patients have at least three different problems that they would like to discuss with their physicians. Once interrupted, however, patients do not usually get the chance to present all their problems to the physician. Physicians who do let their patients complete their opening statements have access to a more complete and accurate list of their patients' problems and experience a significant reduction in the frequency of late-arising problems. Of note, most patients who were allowed to complete their opening statements did so in less than 60 seconds.

FACILITATION

Any comment or behavior on the interviewer's part that encourages the patient to keep talking in an open-ended manner can be considered facilitative. The example given above, "Tell me more about your headaches," is one very effective type of facilitative comment. Another would be a head nod to indicate attention. A comment like "Uh-huh" or "Go on" accomplishes similar ends. Attentive silence can also be facilitative, in that the physician's quiet attention usually encourages the patient to keep talking. Finally, repeating the last few words that the patient has said often invites the patient to keep talking.

Most interviewers do not use facilitation enough. This is a skill that needs to be practiced many times for the interviewer to learn how truly effective it can be. In general, whenever a patient brings up a new problem, the interviewer should use nondirective facilitative interventions (several times) to allow the patient to tell the story in his or her own words in order to provide the most useful and accurate information.

For the purposes of illustration, the same young man with headaches can be considered. The physician can use several facilitating comments and nonverbal responses (such as attentive silence) to encourage the nondirective flow of information.

Physician: Can you tell me some more about the headaches?

Patient: Well, they come on slowly over a period of days and seem to come on only in the hay fever season when my allergies get worse.

Physician: You say they only come in hay fever season?

Patient: Well, I guess I might get a headache in the winter or summer, but this is quite rare. Spring and fall tend to be the time the allergies and the headaches come.

Physician: OK (pause and attentive silence).

Patient: This headache now has gone on for five days and I'm having trouble at work. I don't sleep so well either. These allergies are just getting out of hand.

CLARIFICATION AND DIRECTION

To understand clearly what patients mean to convey and to piece together a coherent narrative of a patient's problem, the physician must make use of clarifying and directive questions. Even during the nondirective phase of the interview, the physician may find the need to interrupt the patient's flow of information to clarify jargon or ambiguities or to direct the process. For example:

Physician: You say the allergies have gotten out of hand. Can you help me understand what you mean when you talk about your allergies?

Patient: Well, every spring and fall I sneeze a lot, and my eyes run and itch. My head feels congested and sometimes hurts.

Physicians may also need to interrupt patients to gain an appreciation for the chronology of the problem. For example:

Physician: Can you tell me when these allergies started?
Patient: I've been having them all my life to some degree, but they seem much worse in the last two or three years.

After such a clarification, the physician can return to open-ended facilitation.

Physician: So they've been getting worse in the last two or three years (pause)?
Patient: Yes. I got married three years ago, changed jobs, and had a baby. My life is different now. I can't seem to get enough rest.

The patient has introduced several new subjects at this point and has come to a natural pause. The patient seems to be waiting for the physician to make a decision about where to direct the interview. The physician can choose to let the patient discuss the changes in his life or to direct the interview back toward the headaches or allergies. At the beginning of an interview, when significant psychosocial factors are raised, it is usually preferable to attend to them, at least briefly. After an initial acknowledgment, if the physician decides to return to the physical symptoms, this can be done with directing comments.

Physician: It sounds like you've been under a great deal of stress lately.
Patient: You can say that again. I just never seem to get time for myself.
Physician: This sounds like it could be a problem in itself. Why don't we talk about the headaches for a few more minutes and then come back to the stress situation.

CHECKING

Checking the story by periodically restating what it seems the patient has said is probably the most important information-gathering skill, and it is the least used.[8] Language is replete with complex meanings that can be easily misinterpreted. Furthermore, physicians often have incorrect information about their patients. A physician's memory may not be accurate, or attention may wander when the patient says something important. It is therefore essential for the physician to check the accuracy of information that is received. This takes only a few seconds, but it is a powerful and important intervention. To continue the example given above, the physician can say something such as this:

Physician: Let me check to see if I understand what you have told me so far. You've been having spring and fall allergies all your life, but these have gotten much worse in the last two or three years since you've been under a lot more stress. You sometimes get headaches with these allergies. The headaches tend to come on slowly and develop over several days. You're having one of these headaches now, and it's getting so bad that you are having trouble at work and sleeping at night.

This type of check by restatement accomplishes multiple important functions. It helps the physician review what has been heard and what needs to be explored more. It allows the physician the opportunity to check the accuracy of what he or she thinks the patient actually said. Checking is reassuring to the patient because he or she realizes the doctor is interested in gaining an accurate understanding of the problem, and this promotes the patient's experience of the physician as interested and caring. It allows the patient the opportunity to clarify any misinformation the physician has developed. Checking facilitates and invites further clarification of the problem by the patient. For all these reasons, checking is one of the most important data-gathering skills available to the physician and should be used frequently in the course of routine interviewing.

Beginning interviewers, in particular, find checking useful because of their own anxiety. There are so many different questions that medical students need to learn that they commonly "freeze" and find it hard to know in which direction they should go. They find it hard to remember what they have just heard as they think about what they must ask next. This common problem for learners has led to the development of a cardinal rule for interviewers who feel lost about where to proceed:

When in doubt, check.

This is a safe, effective, and usually efficient way to get out of trouble. If an interviewer becomes confused, lost, or uncertain of how to proceed, he or she can always say something like this:

Physician: I'd like to take a few moments now to make sure that I have understood you correctly. You told me that . . .

This checking comment invites the patient into a partnership to reconsider the information that has been received. This intervention has proved enormously helpful to beginning students.

Checking helps prevent the painful and embarrassing situation in which a student presents information to a supervisor that may be later contradicted by the patient during the supervisor's interview. Taking the opportunity to check information carefully validates its accuracy and helps to prevent embarrassing situations for learners.

Even experienced physicians can collect inaccurate information from patients. Patients' understanding and recollection of symptoms may develop in an articulate form only during the process of being interviewed. Thus, checking by restatement is an essential skill for experienced interviewers as well as for beginning students.[7]

SURVEYING PROBLEMS: "WHAT ELSE?"

Many interviewing texts do not emphasize the importance of surveying problems. George Engel, an internist, psychoanalyst, and one of the pioneers in the development of medical interviewing, has particularly emphasized this skill.[13] He has stated that he considered, "What else is bothering you?" to be the most important question he asked his patients.

Patients often are anxious or embarrassed about discussing their most serious worries (e.g., "Do I have AIDS?" or "Why am I impotent?") and may leave their chief concern until the end of an interview, when the physician is ready to terminate the session. Sometimes, if the physician guides the interview too strongly, patients are too anxious to remember to discuss all their concerns, or there are simply too many to get to.

The physician should survey problems in the early stages of every interview. It is useful and efficient in the long run for the physician to hear the complete list of the patient's problems before going into a detailed exploration of any of them. This may help prevent a situation, for example, in which a patient's presenting complaint is a headache, but the patient does not mention symptoms of angina-like chest pain until the end of the interview. This type of late-arising or "end-of-the-interview" problem can develop because of patient anxiety about bringing up important symptoms earlier or simply because of patient unawareness of the critical importance of some symptoms. At the end of the interview, for example, the patient may say something like, "Oh, by the way, doctor . . . is this chest pain important?"

Late questions create difficulties for physicians because they are unpredictable, add anxiety, and require time and attention that may not already have been allocated to this patient. Such situations are common; recent studies indicate they occur in up to 20% to 35% of interviews.[12,14] Use of surveying techniques can decrease these problems significantly.

Surveying problems allows the patient and the physician to get an understanding of the medical landscape and then decide which territory to explore first. This increases the efficiency of the interview and allows the patient and physician together to make informed decisions about how to spend the available time.

In practice, it is recommended that the physician begin surveying problems shortly after eliciting and briefly exploring the patient's chief complaint. (The chief complaint is defined as the patient's response to the physician's first open-ended question: "What problem brought you here today?" The chief complaint is reviewed in detail in Chapter 8.) For example:

Physician: Now that I've heard a little about your headache, your allergies, and some of your recent stresses, I'd like to make sure I know something about all your other problems before we get back to them one at a time. What else is bothering you?

"What else is bothering you?" is a more effective question than, "Is there anything else bothering you?" The former question invites the patient to come up with other problems and suggests that the physician is expecting more information from the patient. The latter form is a more closed-ended question and, depending on tone and inflection, can actually be used to cut off discussion. An example might be:

Physician: You don't have any other problems, do you?

Surveying problems should proceed until the patient indicates that there are no other problems. The physician should continue asking, "What else is bothering you?" until the patient indicates that all the problems have been mentioned.

AVOIDING LEADING (BIASED) QUESTIONS

Because of the social power differential in a medical interview, patients tend to be strongly influenced by the wording of a doctor's question, especially if the wording implies that a certain kind of answer is expected. Such a question is called a "leading question." Leading questions can result in significant and sometimes dangerous misinformation, such as in the following example:

Physician: The pain doesn't go down your arm, does it?
Patient: No, not really.

Because the patient usually wants to please the doctor, a leading question will usually elicit the answer the doctor expects. In the example given above, a patient may, in fact, overtly confirm the doctor's expectation that the pain does not go down the arm. This information might not be entirely true, however, as implied by the patient's ambiguous response, "not really."

Sometimes the bias may be less obvious and yet just as powerful. For example, "How helpful was the medication I gave you?" may be a problematic question if the patient thinks the doctor is hoping for a positive response. By adding the phrase, "that I gave you," the physician may link the medication to the person of the doctor in a way that the patient may have difficulty separating. The patient may overemphasize the positive if he or she thinks that is what the doctor wants to hear. Even if the medication had a mixed benefit, if the patient thinks the doctor wants to hear a positive response, the patient may say something like, "It was pretty helpful."

To try and minimize bias, this last question might be rephrased in the following manner:

Physician: What effects, good and bad, did the medication have?

Phrasing the question in this way, the physician can eliminate the bias that might lead the patient to incomplete or inaccurate statements.

CONCLUSION

Gathering accurate data is the central task of patient assessment. Numerous problems exist in the current communication patterns of many physicians: inefficient and ineffective interviewing can lead to misinformation, incomplete information, and frustrating or lengthy visits. Skillful use of basic data-gathering skills such as open-ended questioning, facilitation, and checking can lead to increased efficiency, with improved patient and physician satisfaction and clinical outcome.

REFERENCES

1. Kassirer JP: Teaching clinical medicine by iterative hypothesis testing, *N Engl J Med* 309:921-923, 1983.
2. Elstein A: Psychological research on diagnostic reasoning. In Lipkin M Jr, Putnam SM, Lazare A, editors: *The medical interview: clinical care, education, and research,* New York, 1995, Springer, pp 504-510.
3. Mandin H, Jones A, Woloshuk W, et al: Helping students learn to think like experts when solving clinical problems, *Acad Med* 72:173-179, 1997.
4. Putnam S, Lipkin M Jr: The patient centered interview: research support. In Lipkin M, Putnam SM, Lazare A, editors: *The medical interview: clinical care, education, and research,* New York, 1995, Springer, pp 530-537.
5. Roter DL, Hall JA: Physicians' interviewing styles and medical information obtained from patient, *J Gen Intern Med* 2:325-329, 1987.

6. Maguire P, Faulkner A, Booth K, et al: Helping cancer patients disclose their concern, *Eur J Cancer* 32A:78-81, 1996.
7. Cox A, Rutter M, Holbrook D: Psychiatric interviewing techniques. II. Naturalistic study, *Br J Psychiatry* 138:283-291, 1981.
8. Goldberg D, Steele JJ, Smith C, et al: *Training family practice residents to recognize psychiatric disturbances,* Rockville, Md, 1983, National Institute of Mental Health.
9. Kaplan SH, Greenfield S, Ware JS: Impact of the doctor-patient relationship on the outcome of chronic disease. In Stewart M, Roter D, editors: *Communicating with medical patients,* London, 1989, Sage Publications.
10. Beckman HB, Frankel RM: The effect of physician behavior on the collection of data, *Ann Intern Med* 101:692-696, 1984.
11. Marvel K, Epstein R, Flowers K, et al: Soliciting the patient's agenda: have we improved? *JAMA* 281(3):281-287, 1999.
12. Engel G: Personal communication.
13. White J, Levinson W, Roter D: "Oh, by the way"—the closing moments of the medical interview, *J Gen Intern Med* 9:24-28, 1994.

CHAPTER 5 Function Three: Managing the Patient's Problems (Education, Negotiation, and Motivation)

The third function of the interview concerns the flow of information from the physician to the patient. Patient education is not as simple as it may at first appear. Many factors interfere with the successful transfer of information from the physician to the patient, such as patient anxiety, physician use of overly technical language, patient confusion, and patient misunderstanding. Because of these and other factors, many patients are not well informed about their illnesses and the recommended treatments. Even after physicians believe they have "educated" their patients, the patients have acquired only about 50% of the relevant information.[1] This chapter discusses a few basic communication skills that can considerably enhance physicians' effectiveness as educators.

In the area of overall cooperation with treatment plans, only 22% to 72% of physicians' recommendations are followed. These recommendations include medication adherence, appointment keeping, and life-style alterations (e.g., changes in diet, exercise, or negative habits like smoking). The more acute and life-threatening the illness and the less the amount of change required by the recommendation, the more likely that the patient will follow the advice.[2] There are several simple approaches a physician can take that can dramatically increase the likelihood that a patient will follow his or her advice.[3]

Some might argue that a physician should not be in the business of motivating patients to change. Perhaps physicians should just inform patients of their condition and make recommendations. Perhaps patients should have the right to decide independently whether they want to follow treatment recommendations, without the added burden of physicians' attempts at motivation. While there is certainly some merit to this position, most physicians accept that health enhancement strategies are part of the modern practice of medicine.

Our society is not composed of unrelated, atomistic individuals. The ill health of one individual affects the whole society. Lost work productivity, impaired social and family functioning, and the economic costs of illness all reverberate through society. Furthermore, patients often do not have the perspective of the physician in really understanding the consequences of poor compliance. A young patient with hypertension may not appreciate the real dangers of a stroke, nor can he or she really understand the disability associated with it. Psychologic obstacles or defenses like denial may block a patient from acting in his or her best interests.

There is a continuum of physician activity in the area of influencing patients that ranges from education and influence to motivation and, finally, coercion.[4] Education is the most simple, straightforward, and noncontroversial. In addition, most physicians already try to get their patients to do what they think is best for them. A physician's skill in using motivational strategies to achieve adaptive health behaviors represents another level of activity that most observers consider legitimate.

The more effective the physician is at using motivational strategies, the more power he or she can be said to be exerting over the patient. Thus even the use of motivational strategies may be considered ethically ambiguous because the physician is attempting to influence the patient. Coercion is of course the ultimate type of influence and should rarely be used by a physician. For example, most observers would agree that a psychotic patient refusing antibiotics for life-threatening meningitis should be forced to accept treatment, even against his or her will. In sum, there is a continuum of physician influence from education to coercion, and motivation falls somewhere in between.

This chapter presents a few basic educational and motivational skills that can be used in the general practice of medicine. The physician must exercise clinical and ethical judgment in each case when deciding how much power should be used in each patient encounter. However, it should also be pointed out that the use of even the most up-to-date and skilled motivational interventions does not guarantee success; even the most effective motivator may be ineffectual with some patients at the extreme of nonadherence. (Chapter 22 discusses communication strategies for this group of challenging patients.)

The third function of the interview encompasses a group of important skills that all relate to the physician's efforts to influence the patient's behavior: education about illness, negotiation and maintenance of a treatment plan, and motivation of nonadherent patients. There are three separate sets of skills that relate to each of these related but conceptually and pragmatically distinct areas. These three aspects of patient behavior change will be addressed separately. Previous work by Lazare and colleagues[5] has contributed significantly to the understanding of this function of the interview. Work by Grueninger and associates[6] has helped shape the specific content of the skills.

EDUCATION ABOUT ILLNESS

There are six steps in the process of educating a patient about his or her illness: (1) eliciting the patient's ideas about etiology; (2) providing a basic diagnosis; (3) responding to the patient's feelings about the diagnosis; (4) checking the patient's knowledge of the illness; (5) providing details of the diagnosis; and (6) checking the patient's understanding of the problem.

Eliciting the Patient's Ideas about Etiology

Patients usually have an idea or fear about the cause of their symptoms. It is often most appropriate for physicians to obtain this information at an early stage of the interview process (i.e., as part of the first function of the interview). However, if this information has not been obtained, it is important to obtain these data before attempting to provide the patient with specific diagnostic impressions. By understanding the patient's particular ideas and concerns about his or her illness, the physician will be better able to relieve the patient's anxieties about the illness and respond to the patient's particular concerns.[7] Several studies have shown elicitation of the patient's perspective to be associated with improved clinical outcomes.[8,9]

To obtain the patient's perspective, the physician may find it useful to ask a rather open-ended question such as:

Physician: Patients usually have some ideas or worries about what might be causing their problems. What ideas do you have?

Some patients may be too embarrassed to reveal their fears, and encouragement from the physician may be necessary. For example:

Patient: I don't know what could be causing this. That's why I came to you. You're the doctor.

Physician: You're right. I am the doctor, and I will do what I can to figure out the problem and help you with it. But most patients do have certain ideas or fears about their problems, like whether this is cancer, or whether this is diabetes. If you've had some ideas or worries, I'd like to know about them, so I can be of more help to you.

At this point, many patients will admit to fears about particular illnesses that they dread, that they may have read about, or with which they have had particular experiences. Such common illnesses as cancer, heart disease, and dementia often frighten patients. If the physician is aware of these fears, the patient can be saved considerable anxiety. The physician can increase overall interviewing efficiency by addressing these fears right away.

Providing a Basic Diagnosis

After the physician addresses the patient's basic concerns or fears, the patient should be provided with the basic diagnostic information. It is important to give this information briefly and succinctly. The patient will be very anxious while listening to diagnostic information, and he or she will not be able to understand or remember much information that is not delivered in short, discrete bundles. One or two sentences should be all that is said in providing the basic diagnosis. For example:

> **Physician:** Mr. Brown, you have diabetes.
> *or*
> Mrs. Jones, you have high blood pressure.

These short sentences are sufficient for the first piece of information. The patient will then have some more specific questions or will demonstrate some emotional response.

Giving bad news is far more delicate and complicated, but it also should be short and succinct. This particular communication challenge is discussed in more detail in Chapter 24. It is usually best to include some hopeful statement along with the bad news. Despite the gravity of the condition, some general comment indicating continued attention should be made. For example:

> **Physician:** Mr. Wright, I'm sorry to have to tell you that you have cancer of the colon. It is serious, but I want you to be sure to understand that there is a lot we can do for you.

Responding to the Patient's Feelings about the Diagnosis

Patients will often respond emotionally to news about the diagnosis of their conditions. This is particularly true if they are receiving bad news. At times, this response may be only nonverbal. They may become especially silent and look sad, fearful, or anxious. They may weep or ask a lot of questions.

The physician should make it clear to the patient that the expression of feelings is acceptable and understandable. Physician statements of reflection and legitimation are usually appropriate here, as is nonverbal support such as attentive silence or holding the patient's hand. If the patient has just heard bad news, the physician should provide realistic hope along with emotional support. For the patient who is visibly shaken, the physician can say something like:

> **Physician:** I see how upsetting this news is for you. I'm going to do everything I can to help you through this and I'm going to be here for you personally as well. I want you to remember that there's a lot we can do to fight this thing together.

Even when a diagnosis is not immediately life threatening, the patient often has an emotional reaction that should be acknowledged by the physician. By acknowledging this emotion, the physician allows the patient to verbalize particular fears about the illness. This will ultimately increase efficiency in the interview and enable the physician to better support the patient.

Checking the Patient's Knowledge of the Illness

Many patients already know a great deal about their illness. Unless the physician actually inquires about this knowledge, a great deal of time may be wasted by telling the patient something he or she already knows. Patients may also have a great deal of misinformation. If this is elicited early in the interview, it can be corrected before it has a deleterious effect. The physician can say something like:

> **Physician:** Before I go into more details about high blood pressure, what causes it and what can happen if we don't control it, perhaps you can tell me what you already know about high blood pressure and its treatment.

Providing Details of the Diagnosis

After the physician has provided the basic diagnosis, responded to the patient's emotions, and established the patient's baseline knowledge, the physician can elaborate on the details of the diagnosis. The physician should take pains to use language that the patient will understand and use short sentences that make the point very clearly. The physician should stop frequently to check the patient's understanding and ask for questions, as described in the next section.

Checking the Patient's Understanding of the Problem

Checking patient understanding is the physician's most important educational skill. A physician cannot be sure that a patient understands what he or she has been told unless the physician checks. For example, the physician can say:

> **Physician:** I would like to make sure that I have been able to make this information clear. Would you mind telling me what you understand about your condition?

Similarly, after the patient has demonstrated appropriate understanding, the physician should check what questions the patient has about the illness:

> **Physician:** What questions do you have about what we discussed?

This question is most useful if it is presented in this positive manner, assuming that the patient does have questions. If the physician asks, "Do you have any questions?" the patient may respond, "No," simply out of social embarrassment.

NEGOTIATION AND MAINTENANCE OF A TREATMENT PLAN

Once the physician has reviewed the important diagnostic information and has responded to the patient's emotional reactions to the diagnostic news, the physician must negotiate a treatment plan with the patient and take steps to maintain this plan. There are seven basic steps to the negotiation and maintenance of a treatment plan: (1) checking baseline information; (2) describing treatment goals (with options, if any) and treatment plans (with options, if any); (3) checking understanding; (4) eliciting patient preferences and commitments; (5) negotiating a plan cooperatively; (6) eliciting specific patient affirmation of intent; and (7) planning for maintenance and relapse prevention.

Checking Baseline Information

Before the physician begins to describe treatment options, he or she should determine what the patient already knows or believes about treatment. Some or all of this information may have already been provided when the doctor asked about the patient's baseline information of the illness (see Checking the Patient's Knowledge of the Illness).

Describing Treatment Goals and Plans (With Options, If Any)

For many chronic illnesses, there is a range of treatment goals and interventions that can be selected. The physician should review these options with the patient. If there is only one reasonable treatment strategy (e.g., antibiotics for an acute infection), the physician should also make this clear at this time. For example, with hypertension, the goals can vary considerably, from losing weight and getting more exercise to taking pills regularly and changing the salt content of the diet, among other options. The physician should describe these options clearly and succinctly.

Checking Understanding

For chronic illnesses with a range of treatment options, the physician should make sure that the patient understands the different possibilities presented. The physician can say something like:

> **Physician:** I would like to make sure that I have been able to communicate the treatment possibilities to you clearly. Would you mind reviewing your understanding of these options now?

Eliciting Patient Preferences and Commitments

Once the patient has clearly understood the range of options that are possible, the physician should ask the patient what he or she is willing to do. For example:

> **Physician:** Now that we have reviewed the treatment options, what would you like to do about your high blood pressure? How can I be of help to you?

Negotiating a Plan Cooperatively; Anticipating Problems and Solutions

The patient's desires and intentions will often differ from the physician's recommendation. The development of a treatment plan must therefore be negotiated with the patient. Each part of the plan must be worked out in very explicit detail so that it is clear to both the patient and the physician what is being agreed upon. Once the plan has been described (and preferably written down), it is important to anticipate problems and find solutions. In the anticipation of problems, it is generally better to ask the patient to anticipate problems and then ask the patient to think of possible solutions. Typical problems include such things as forgetting medication and overeating. If the patient can come up with ideas for resolving problems himself or herself, the chances of success will be greater.

However, if patients do not mention common problems like forgetting or side effects, the doctor should mention them. Sometimes the patient does not or cannot come up with ideas to overcome these obstacles. In such cases, the physician can present ideas that have often worked for others (e.g., involving significant others in the plan, using memory aids, scheduling frequent follow-up visits, or using self-motivating strategies). In addition, providing appropriate reading materials, referring the patient to appropriate and available health educators, and teaching specific skills would all be relevant interventions at this point.

Eliciting Specific Patient Affirmation of Intent

After the plan has been developed, having the patient review the intentions explicitly is usually helpful and increases the chances of accurate adherence.[10] The physician can ask the patient to state specific plans:

> **Physician:** Now that we have arrived at a plan, would you mind letting me know very specifically what you plan to do to help with the high blood pressure?

Planning for Maintenance and Prevention of Relapse

It is not enough to embark successfully on an initial treatment plan. Many patients will become nonadherent over time if they are not part of an active maintenance program to prevent relapse. This usually requires frequent follow-up visits (or contacts) to check the patient's adherence to the behavioral plan. Follow-up visits must involve careful checking of adherence and an attempt to resolve any problems the patient may be having with the treatment program.

MOTIVATION

Many patients seem to understand their illness and its treatment, yet have trouble adhering to a management plan. Overall, between 22% and 72% of patients do not adhere to the medication or other recommendations of their physicians. The highest rates of nonadherence occur with respect to suggestions for life-style modifications. These include suggestions such as stopping smoking, altering the diet, obtaining regular exercise, and following through on mammography recommendations.

There are seven steps in a basic motivational sequence that physicians can use to help motivate patients to adhere to treatment plans. (Chapter 22 presents a higher-order framework for dealing with motivation and patient behavior change in medical practice.) The seven basic steps are particularly important to adopt for patients who are recognized by physicians as at least partially nonadherent to treatment plans. Depending on the severity of the clinical situation, some of these steps can be abbreviated or omitted. The steps are as follows: (1) checking adherence carefully; (2) diagnosing specific adherence problems; (3) responding to emotions and offering support, partnership, and respect; (4) eliciting personal preferences and a statement of commitment; (5) negotiating solutions; (6) obtaining an affirmation of intent and follow-up; and (7) responding to emotions throughout.

Checking Adherence Carefully (Nonjudgmental, Open Ended)

To check adherence carefully, the physician should help patients admit to the problems they may be having without causing them embarrassment or humiliation. If doctors ask their patients something like, "Have you been taking your medication?" many patients will be too embarrassed to answer the question honestly. A less judgmental and more open-ended and productive way to inquire about adherence is something like:

Physician: Most patients have trouble keeping up with their medications. What trouble have you been having taking your medications regularly?[11]

Given this opening to admit difficulties, many patients will be more willing to admit to the truth. Some patients remain hesitant to discuss nonadherence and say something like:

Patient: I haven't had any difficulties.

The physician can then continue to explore nonadherence by saying something like:

> **Physician:** Well, if you've had no trouble, that's great. But most of my patients do have some troubles. I would really like to hear if you've had any difficulties at all, no matter how minor.

Again, given this type of permission, many patients will be more likely to discuss their problems openly.

Diagnosing Specific Adherence Problems

Once patients have indicated that there may be some difficulties in maintaining the treatment plan, the physician should attempt to clarify the specific problems that exist. The most common difficulties with taking medication on schedule are forgetting and side effects. Problems with understanding the program can also cause treatment nonadherence. The following sequence of questions is often useful in clarifying the specific adherence problems:

> **Physician:** Can you review for me, in detail, what your understanding of the treatment plan has been?
> **Physician:** What have you actually been able to do?
> **Physician:** What kinds of problems have arisen to make it difficult to follow the treatment plan?

Difficulties with life-style changes usually relate to problems with motivation and commitment. When dealing with significant motivational problems, physicians should remember that some patients are simply not ready for or interested in following treatment recommendations. This problem is discussed at length in Chapter 22 on managing the nonadherent patient. For general purposes, however, physicians should understand that some patients will not even contemplate the possibility of change. Prochaska and DiClemente[12] have termed this position the "precontemplation" stage of change. To determine whether the patient is in the precontemplation stage, the physician must ask the patient directly and nonjudgmentally. For example:

> **Physician:** It seems to me that you are really not interested or able to consider stopping smoking at this time.

If the patient makes it clear that he or she is not ready to consider stopping smoking (or stopping drinking, or losing weight, etc.), the physician should accept this position without a blaming attitude. Judging the patient will usually push the patient away and will not help him or her eventually change a negative health habit. Furthermore, the physician should not waste time, energy, and emotion in fruitless motivational appeals toward a patient who is essentially in the precontemplative position. Only when the patient indicates his or her own genuine personal interest in changing a behavior (stage of contemplation) can the physician help the patient develop a workable plan.

For patients in precontemplation, the key interventions the physician can make center on attempting to move the patient to a stage of reflection or contemplation about change. One vehicle for this can be to ensure that the patient understands the health consequences of his or her own behavior.

For patients who are genuinely contemplating change and for whom the specific adherence problems have been clarified, it is then possible for the physician and patient to develop a plan together to address the problems.

Responding to Emotions: Offering Support, Partnership, and Respect

When the patient begins telling the physician about his or her difficulties, the physician should indicate an understanding of the problem and legitimate the patient's feelings. For example:

Physician: I get the feeling that you don't like this low-salt diet.
Patient: I hate it. The food has no taste.
Physician: I can see that this is a real problem for you. A lot of patients have the same problem.

An offer of support can be helpful:

Physician: I want you to know that I will do whatever I can to help you work this problem out.

Similarly, an offer of partnership often sets a tone conducive to effective collaboration and exploration.

Physician: I realize that the low-salt diet is a real problem for you. Perhaps if you and I put our heads together, we might come up with some ideas that could help you reach your goals.

It is important that the physician respects or praises whatever the patient has already successfully accomplished. For example:

Physician: I'm impressed that you've been able to stick to the diet even a little, given the fact that you dislike it so much.

Eliciting Personal Preferences and a Statement of Commitment

For the patient and physician to develop a new plan, it is important for the patient to be able to make a commitment to try again. Before directly asking the patient to state his or her preferences and to make a commitment, it is usually helpful for the physician to comment explicitly on the patient's characteristics that might help the physician and patient plan together. In addition, the focus should be on helping the patient develop his or her own autonomous choices. Research indicates that the likelihood of adherence is much higher if the patient produces the idea himself or herself than if the physician suggests the plan.[13]

For example, the physician might say:

> **Physician:** We have reviewed some of the difficulties you have been having in keeping to the treatment plan. This is certainly no easy task. On the other hand, it is clear to me that you are quite knowledgeable about your illness and also that you are concerned about your health. What are you willing to do at this point?

At times, appeals to other values such as responsibility, family, or danger of ill health might be helpful in eliciting a statement of commitment.

If the patient indicates that he or she is willing or interested in trying to develop a new treatment program, the physician can proceed with the other steps in the motivation sequence. Keeping the focus on the patient's own ideas is extremely important and can help in developing practical solutions.

Negotiating Solutions

Once the patient has indicated a willingness to try again, the physician should begin by eliciting the patient's own ideas about a new program that might work. For example, the physician could say:

> **Physician:** I'm wondering what ideas you might have that might help you remember to take the pills more regularly.

Patients will be much more likely to adhere to a plan to which they have contributed than to one that is offered by the physician without their own participation.

If patients develop ideas that seem to have a likelihood of success, the physician should respect these ideas and work out the specifics of the program in detail. At times, it may be necessary for the physician to offer a range of ideas. The physician might say something like:

> **Physician:** Let me tell you a few ideas that have worked for other patients. Perhaps one of them might be something you'd like to try.

The most common ideas include involving the patient's support system in the treatment program, tailoring the medication to daily habit schedules, scheduling frequent follow-ups, self-monitoring, and developing small, manageable, realistic goals.

The patient may propose ideas that are unrealistic or not medically sound. For example:

Patient: I guess I will just have to skip this low-salt deal.

The patient may also propose ideas that are not likely to be effective, such as:

Patient: I guess I will just have to try harder.

The physician must tactfully point out the problems. The physician can say:

Physician: Well, I really wish we could skip the diet problems, but it is important to remember that the level of your salt intake really does represent a significant risk to your health.

Or similarly, a physician might say:

Physician: Trying harder is a reasonable idea, but it seems to me that just trying harder didn't work before, and it might not work again. Do you have any more specific ideas that might help you cut down on your salt intake?

When the patient develops an adaptive idea that seems likely to succeed, the physician should respect the idea and indicate appreciation. For example:

Physician: I think your idea of limiting salt to one meal a day is an excellent idea. Which meal will that be, and how much salt do you plan to use at that meal?

In general, the more concrete and specific the program, the more likely it will be to succeed.

Once an adherence plan has been mutually developed and negotiated, the physician should explore possible problems with the patient. For example:

Physician: Now that you have decided to limit your salt intake to your evening meal and will ask your wife to put only a small amount of salt on your vegetables, what kind of problem do you anticipate in keeping to this program?

When the patient indicates some specific problems that might develop, the physician should return to step 3 and ask the patient to develop his or her own ideas again about adaptive strategies to deal with these possible problems. It should be clear that the process of negotiating an effective treatment plan that has a reasonable chance of success with a previously nonadherent patient could be time consuming. The greatest amount of time is used in eliciting very specific behavioral plans directly from the patient. Understanding that this process takes some time to succeed can help physicians plan appropriately. The investment in time is well worth the effort.

Obtaining an Affirmation of Intent and Follow-up

Once the plan has been established, the physician should ask the patient to review the plan and state his or her specific intentions. For example, the physician might say:

Physician: Just to make sure we understand each other, would you mind reviewing with me now what you plan to do about your treatment?

Definite plans for follow-up and adherence monitoring must be established at this point. For example:

Physician: That sounds like an excellent plan. I'd like for you to come back next week and let me know how things have been going with respect to the treatment plan.

Responding to Emotions Throughout

Most motivational efforts will arouse emotions in the patient. These include anxiety, sadness, anger, humiliation, happiness, and sadness. These emotions may often impede the educational or motivational process.

Whenever the physician notices an emotion, particularly if it interferes with the negotiation, he or she should return to rapport- and relationship-building skills and respond to the patient's emotions. For example, if the patient becomes quiet and sullen, the physician should say something like:

Physician: Something seems to be bothering you now about what we're doing.

This type of comment will usually encourage the patient to discuss the feelings that are troubling. If the patient becomes anxious, the physician can add:

Physician: I see that this discussion seems to be making you a little nervous. Can you tell me something about that?

CONCLUSION

Efficient and effective patient education, negotiation, and motivation require the use of complex skills of utmost importance for ensuring optimal patient outcome. The interventions outlined above, however, represent basic, pragmatic approaches that can be effective for most patients. These interventions provide structures for physicians to use for educating their routine patients, as well as outlines of how to approach their more difficult, nonadherent patients.

REFERENCES

1. Stewart M: Patient recall and comprehension after the medical visit. In Lipkin M Jr, Putnam SM, Lazare A, editors: *The medical interview: clinical care, education, and research,* New York, 1995, Springer, pp 525-529.
2. Sackett DL, Snow JC: The magnitude of compliance and noncompliance. In Haynes R, Taylor D, Sackett DL, editors: *Compliance in health care,* Baltimore, 1979, Johns Hopkins University Press.
3. Meichenbaum D, Turk DC: *Facilitating treatment adherence,* New York, 1987, Plenum Press.
4. Tomlinson T: The physicians' influence on patients' choices, *Theoret Med* 7:105-121, 1986.
5. Lazare A, Putnam SM, Lipkin M Jr: Three functions of the medical interview. In Lipkin M Jr, Putnam SM, Lazare A, editors: *The medical interview: clinical care, education, and research,* New York, 1995, Springer, pp 3-19.
6. Grueninger U, Duffy DF, Goldstein M: Patient education in the medical encounter: how to facilitate learning, behavior change, and coping. In Lipkin M Jr, Putnam SM, Lazare A, editors: *The medical interview: clinical care, education, and research,* New York, 1995, Springer, pp 122-133.
7. Stewart MA, Belle Brown J, Wayne Weston W, et al: *Patient-centered medicine: transforming the clinical method,* Thousand Oaks, Calif, 1995, Sage.
8. Orth JE, Stiles WB, Scherwitz L, et al: Patient exposition and provider explanation in routine interviews and hypertensive patients' blood pressure control, *Health Psychol* 6:29-42, 1987.
9. Henbest RJ, Stewart M: Patient-centeredness in the consultation. 2. Does it really make a difference? *Fam Pract* 7:28-33, 1990.

10. Dye N, DiMatteo MR: Enhancing cooperation with the medial regimen. In Lipkin M Jr, Putnam SM, Lazare A, editors: *The medical interview: clinical care, education, and research,* New York, 1995, Springer, pp 134-146.
11. Haynes R, Taylor D, Sackett DL, editors: *Compliance in health care,* Baltimore, 1979, Johns Hopkins University Press.
12. Prochaska JO, DiClemente CC: Towards a comprehensive model of change. In Miller R, Heather N, editors: *Treating addictive behaviors,* New York, 1986, Plenum Press.
13. Dye N, DiMatteo MR: Enhancing cooperation with the medical regimen. In Lipkin M Jr, Putnam SM, Lazare A, editors: *The medical interview: clinical care, education, and research,* New York, 1995, Springer, pp 134-146.

UNIT

II

MEETING THE PATIENT

CHAPTER

6 Ten Common Concerns

Most medical students eagerly anticipate their first contacts with patients. Many students spend at least 1 year, and sometimes beyond that, in classroom settings before they ever get a chance to talk with a patient. Therefore, courses on clinical methods, physical diagnoses, or the doctor-patient relationship usually come as a great relief to students because they may be finally getting a taste of what "real" medicine will be like for them. Most physicians remember their first interviews with patients well because these early encounters mark the beginnings of their careers in a real, as well as symbolic, way. These first contacts with patients are some of the most exciting and moving aspects of medical education.

Along with reasonable and expected excitement comes anxiety. Medical students are almost always anxious before they meet their first patients. The sources of this anxiety are numerous and understandable. Students may feel worried about how the patients will react to them. They are usually concerned that the patients will feel intruded upon. They imagine that the interview will invade the patients' privacy and dignity.

Worse than medical students' concern about invading patients' privacy during an interview is concern about another part of the students' education. When students are learning the basic elements of the physical examination, they must impose upon the patient to be exposed physically and sometimes to undergo painful examination. Some students view this as another indignity and humiliation to the patient. Students often ask themselves, "Why must the patient go through this, just for my education?" These concerns become more intense if the patient is seriously ill or dying.

The student who feels anxious about interviewing patients should be assured that he or she is in good company. Learning to interview involves learning not only a new set of difficult and complex skills, but also the assumption of a new and dramatically different social role. In putting on the white coat for the first time, the student automatically attains the social status of a physician. This simple, symbolic dressing change signifies a momentous interpersonal change. Suddenly, the student is required to ask intimate questions of other people and to tell other people to undress and be examined. Even stranger to some students is that these other people (patients) usually do what they are told and treat the students with enormous respect.

Learning to function in the new and powerful social role of the physician understandably makes most medical students anxious. There are many questions students ask themselves and their instructors as they begin this part of their training. Ten common concerns are discussed in this chapter.

1. Why should the patient want to talk to or be examined by a student?
2. Is a student interview or examination a humiliation or indignity for the patient?
3. How should I dress? Should I wear a white coat?
4. Should I introduce myself as "doctor"? If I do that, am I not deceiving the patient?
5. If the patient is in pain or emotional distress, should I continue with the interview?
6. Should I shake the patient's hand? Under what circumstances is it acceptable to touch a patient?
7. If the patient asks me questions, should I answer the questions if I know the answers? What should I do if I do not know the answers?
8. What do I do if the patient starts crying or if the patient gets angry with me?
9. What should I do if the patient tells me something his or her doctor does not know? For example, what if the patient tells me that he or she is depressed or suicidal?
10. What should I do if the patient promises to tell me some important secrets if I agree to maintain his or her confidence?

Why Should the Patient Want to Talk to or Be Examined by a Student?

Students usually find it difficult to understand the reasons that a patient should want to be interviewed by a student or, even worse, to be examined by a student. Students may wonder what the patient could possibly gain from this encounter.

Most patients are willing to be interviewed and examined by students. Patients usually understand that students need to learn about illness with real patients, and patients often derive altruistic satisfaction from allowing themselves to be such subjects. Patients rarely feel like guinea pigs. More commonly, patients interviewed or examined by medical students feel that they are making a genuine and active contribution by assisting in the training of physicians. Participating in such educational activities often plays a profound and critical role in the psychologic adaptation of the severely ill or incapacitated. The feelings of uselessness that are associated with illness can be meaningfully counteracted for some patients by their sense of contribution to the education of future physicians. Thus even if students do nothing else positive for patients, patients may benefit from the interview and physical examination by being allowed to "give" something to physicians in training.

Most students do give patients something important. The concern, interest, and attention provided by the student can offer significant emotional comfort to the patient. Although it is sometimes intangible and difficult to measure, this emotional dimension to the student-patient interaction can be dramatic. Patients often interpret even the physical examination as an emotional gift. Thus students would do well to realize that most patients are willing and even eager to be interviewed and examined.

Of course, some patients do not want to be interviewed or examined. Before beginning, students need to ask patients if they are willing to be interviewed. If the patients indicate that they do not want to be interviewed, these wishes must be respected. In these situations the students should politely thank the patients and leave. The students should check with their supervisors for guidance in how to proceed further.

Is a Student Interview or Examination a Humiliation or Indignity for the Patient?

Some students feel awkward because they think patients will feel humiliated when subjecting themselves to an interview by a student. Students have this fear partly because of the implied power of the role of the physician. Students feel uncomfortable assuming this power when they "do not deserve it" because they are not able to offer true medical assistance. As pointed out previously, however, few patients feel this embarrassment or humiliation.

How Should I Dress? Should I Wear a White Coat Even Though I Am Not a Doctor? Doesn't This Introduce an Artificial Separation and Inequality into the Relationship? If I Wear a White Coat, Isn't That Deceiving the Patient?

In general, students should dress in the same attire as the other physicians in their institution. If most of the other doctors wear whites, students should wear whites. Dressing in the same manner as the physicians indicates respect for the patient.

Dressing as a physician distinguishes students from patients and introduces an inequality into the student-patient relationship. This distinction and inequality are both appropriate. Students will be interviewing patients and asking them to divulge some of the most intimate details of their lives. Patients will be asked to undress and to allow themselves to be physically examined. These requests are accepted and expected parts of the doctor-patient relationship.

As discussed in the next section, students should clearly introduce themselves as "student" doctors. This helps ensure that patients will not be deceived.

Should I Introduce Myself as "Doctor"? If I Do, Am I Deceiving the Patient?

Most beginning students are uncomfortable with introducing themselves as "doctor." This discomfort is understandable because many patients do not understand the differences among students, interns, residents, and attending physicians. Students should almost always make their status and level of training clear. The following examples illustrate ways this can be achieved:

> **Student:** Hello. My name is John Smith. I am a medical student taking a course on how to interview patients. I was given your name as someone who might be willing to talk with me about your illness. Would that be all right with you?

Another alternative, for students in a clerkship situation, could be to say something like the following:

> **Student:** Hello. My name is Bill Stevens, and I am a student doctor working with Dr. Jones. Do you mind if I ask you a few questions about your problems before you see Dr. Jones?

In practice, this type of introduction works easily and well for most students and their patients. Patients, on the other hand, often wonder how they should address medical students. Is it appropriate for patients to call the student "doctor," or should patients use a student's first name? There is no clearly appropriate label that conveys the character of the student physician-patient relationship. Most such relationships closely resemble true doctor-patient relationships. They resemble such relationships much more closely than they resemble anything else. Thus it is no surprise that most patients prefer to address their student doctors as "doctor." This is perfectly appropriate, especially if the patient understands that the student is not a licensed physician. Sometimes patients ask students what they want to be called. It is common for students to want to be called by their first names and acceptable in these cases for patients to do so. Similarly, some students prefer to leave this choice to the patients. However, if students would like to be called "doctor," patients can be told something such as the following:

> **Student:** I am a student doctor now and would prefer for you to call me "Doctor Jones." I will be finished with my training in another year. I hope this is acceptable to you.

If the Patient Is in Pain or Emotional Distress, Should I Continue With the Interview?

If the patient is in pain or emotional distress, the wishes of the patient must be respected. First, the student must acknowledge the pain or distress. The student may say something like the following:

> **Student:** You seem to be in distress.
> *or*
> You seem to be in a lot of pain right now.

These comments are appropriate and will let the patient know that his or her suffering has been noticed. Students can and should directly ask whether anything can be done to help. Often patients appreciate a glass of water, a change of the position of the bed, or some other small intervention.

After discomfort has been acknowledged and offers of assistance have been made, the student should ask the patient whether the interview can be conducted or should be postponed. If the patient wants the student to go away, this desire should be respected. Most often and to the surprise of most students, the patient wants to continue the interview or examination. Once pain or distress has been acknowledged, the patient will usually feel comforted by the concern and attention of the student and will prefer to continue.

Should I Shake the Patient's Hand? Under What Circumstances Is It Acceptable to Touch the Patient?

Most physicians offer a hand to their patients in greeting when they introduce themselves. This practice generally works well for beginning students. However, some male students express discomfort with this practice because they have been taught that it is rude to offer a hand to a woman, even for a social or professional greeting. These students have been taught that respectful behavior requires a gentleman to wait for a woman to offer him her hand before he attempts to shake hands. Students who are uncomfortable with shaking hands in greeting will do better to wait for patients to offer a hand to them. Students who are uncomfortable about touching a patient in any way are better advised to avoid the touch than to force themselves into physical contact out of a belief that it may be good for the patient.

Touch is a powerful and supportive technique in medicine. In situations of great distress, physicians commonly and appropriately hold a patient's hand or put an arm around a patient's shoulders. Experienced physicians routinely use measured physical contact to reassure their patients and enhance rapport. Most patients like to be touched appropriately. However, some patients do not want to be touched, and some physicians find that any type of touch (other than the physical examination) provokes anxiety. In general, students and physicians should adhere to the following rule:

> ***If a student feels uncomfortable in touching a patient, this should not be done.***

Discomfort with touching communicates itself to patients through nonverbal channels, and such a touch becomes an anxiety-producing intervention for the patient rather than a support.

Some students and physicians are overly familiar with their patients and touch them too much. Observing the patient is critical. A patient who is uncomfortable with being touched will give some signal, usually nonverbal, that the touch is not appreciated. For example, he or she will back away, stiffen up, or become quiet. The doctor must be vigilant to watch for these signs and respond to them appropriately, generally by backing away respectfully.

Touch can be emotionally or sexually seductive. Physicians should be aware of the tremendous power they wield over their patients. Illness causes patients to regress psychologically and physically and thus elevates the role of the physician in patients' minds. The resulting emotional dependency on the physician is commonly overwhelming. Often, patients are not able to use their most rational thought processes; patients in this situation may relate to their physicians as children relate to their parents. Inappropriate touch can be part of an emotionally seductive doctor-patient relationship that can harm patients by fostering dependency rather than adaptive coping.

Sexual seductiveness can be communicated by touching patients. Tragically, this can lead to sexual relationships between physicians and patients. Because of the grossly unequal power in the doctor-patient relationship and the psychologic dependency of the illness situation, patients may not be able to make mature decisions about sexuality with their physicians. Students and physicians must remember the following ethical principle:

> ***A sexual relationship between a doctor and his or her patient is* ALWAYS *an abuse of power in the doctor-patient relationship. This is exploitative and unethical behavior.***

If the Patient Asks Me Questions, Should I Answer Them if I Know the Answers? What Should I Do If I Do Not Know the Answers?

In general, medical students practicing an interview or physical examination with someone else's patients should avoid answering any questions about a patient's individual condition. In the heady moments of finally being regarded as an expert, students might be tempted to answer some medical question that they think they understand well. It is important to resist this temptation. Students may have an incomplete understanding of the medical issue or may not understand the personal meaning of the question to the patients they are interviewing or examining. Since the students will breeze into and out of the patients' lives in a few hours, the students will not be able to observe the impact of whatever information they give the patients. Some seemingly innocuous question might have great import for the patients. The following statement is important for medical students practicing an interview:

> ***All medical questions should be referred back to the patient's primary physician.***

This rule does not necessarily hold for patients of medical students who are serving clinical clerkships. Such students often become the patients' primary source of information. When students assume the role of educators, however, they should be confident of the information they give to their patients and sensitive to the emotional impact of the information they transmit. Any uncertainty should be reviewed carefully with supervisors.

What Do I Do if the Patient Starts Crying or if the Patient Becomes Angry With Me?

Nothing makes some students (and sometimes physicians) more uncomfortable than the expression of emotion by patients. What should students do when patients start crying? This will be a common occurrence, and students need to start learning how to respond in a way that is helpful and supportive to patients.

An attitude of interest and respect will almost always be comforting to patients, regardless of what the students do or say. Students can communicate this respect and caring nonverbally without any conscious effort. Most patients feel supported and reassured by physicians who can accept and respond appropriately to the limited ventilation of feelings.

Some students and physicians are so uncomfortable with sadness that they communicate their own anxiety to patients. This discomfort is usually interpreted by patients as meaning that the doctors do not want the patients to show any more emotion. Patients usually honor this perception and "cooperate" with their physicians by suppressing the expression of further emotion.

When students have some verbal strategy in mind to deal with situations in which patients are anxious, the students' own anxiety will be less and the students will be able to help patients more. The following general rule has proved useful:

> ***When in doubt about how to respond to a patient's emotions, use reflection and legitimation.***

Comments like the following are appropriate:

> **Student:** I can see that you are very upset by this situation.
> *or*
> I understand this is very troubling.

In general, such reflective comments encourage patients to discuss some details of the troubling situation. This information can usually be followed by legitimating comments such as the following:

> **Student:** I can certainly understand why this has taken such a toll on you.
> *or*
> Anyone would have trouble dealing with this.

What about when patients get angry? This is even more difficult to manage. The natural responses to anger are to withdraw or attack. Neither response is particularly helpful in developing a rapport with angry patients. Of more help is reflection, even of an angry emotion. For example, students can say something such as the following:

> **Student:** This conversation seems to irritate you.

Again, this type of reflective comment will usually lead patients to discuss more of the particular details of their situations. Subsequent to this discussion a legitimating comment may be appropriate:

> **Student:** I can certainly understand why this situation has made you so frustrated.

This difficult topic will be discussed further in Chapter 16.

What Should I Do if the Patient Tells Me Something His or Her Doctor Does Not Know? For Example, What if the Patient Tells Me that He or She Is Depressed or Suicidal?

Because medical students are often deeply interested in their patients and often have more listening time than do the patients' doctors, it is not uncommon for patients to confide levels of psychic distress to students that they have not been able to confide to their own doctors.

> ***This information must always be communicated to the patients' physicians by the students themselves.***

Students can advise patients to tell their physicians directly, but this is not sufficient. If the patients have not already told their physicians, they cannot be relied on to tell their physicians the problems they have discussed with the student doctor. The only way students can be sure that the physicians will become aware of the problem is to tell the physicians themselves.

What Should I Do if the Patient Promises to Tell Me Some Secret if I Agree to Maintain His or Her Confidence?

Since most students demonstrate a high degree of emotional interest in their patients, an occasional patient wants to share some secret that he or she may not want to be shared with the rest of the medical team.

Students should never promise a patient absolute confidentiality.

If a patient asks for confidentiality, the student should indicate that his or her student status makes it impossible to give a promise of complete confidentiality. The student may have to share this information with a supervisor or the patient's treatment team. The student can guarantee to use his or her best judgment about whether any information the patient provides might have relevance to the medical situation. If the student feels the information is relevant to the medical care, he or she must receive supervision from some superior to make sure the information is used appropriately by the medical team.

In general, requests for complete confidentiality represent opportunities for students to enhance the care a patient receives as long as the patient is told the limits of the confidentiality and the information is appropriately handled after it has been received.

UNIT

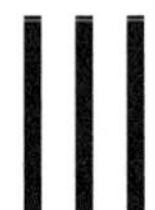

STRUCTURE OF THE INTERVIEW

CHAPTER

7 Opening

The next eight chapters review traditional structural elements of the medical interview. Despite this emphasis on structural elements, the student should remember that each of the three functions of the interview may be used appropriately during any particular phase or structure of the interview, depending on the condition of the patient and the topics being discussed. For example, when reviewing information about the patient's family medical history (function two), if a patient breaks down in tears when discussing his or her parent's death, the interviewer should take time to respond appropriately to the emotions revealed at that moment (function one). Similarly, during the physical examination, a patient may ask a question about moles on the skin, and the physician may find it appropriate to provide education at that point (function three).

To deal systematically with the wealth of information to collect and to both give and build emotional rapport, the skilled physician needs to maintain a rough organizational plan for the interview, which will cover all the relevant structural and functional elements. As described by Lipkin et al,[1] the specific dynamic interaction of each patient and physician with the particularities of the medical condition requires the interviewer to weave a complicated mosaic of both structural elements and functional interventions to achieve all the goals of the interview. This chapter discusses the beginning structure of the encounter between the patient and the physician.

The opening of the interview can be broken into five components. There are of course many different ways a skilled clinician can open an interview with a patient. The following format represents just one approach that is usually effective in laying the groundwork for a therapeutic doctor-patient encounter.

INTRODUCTION

The nonverbal greeting occurs before the actual verbal introduction. The doctor or student should establish good eye contact and (most commonly) extend a friendly hand in greeting. The verbal message follows. For example:

> **Student:** Good morning, Mr. Cummings. My name is Bill Sams. I am a student doctor.

ESTABLISHING GOALS OF THE INTERVIEW

In general, effective interviews begin with an explicit statement or acknowledgment of goals. Sometimes these may need to be negotiated between the doctor and the patient if their objectives differ. For the purposes of the student in a clinical methods class, there needs to be a brief statement about the purposes and the expectations for the interview. This can be done in many ways. For example:

> **Student:** Good morning, Mr. Cummings. My name is Bill Sams, and I am a student doctor learning how to interview patients. Your doctor gave me your name.

OBTAINING PATIENT CONSENT TO YOUR INTERVIEW PLAN

For most interviews in actual practice, patient consent is implied by the patient's presence in the physician's office or hospital. However, in some situations explicit patient consent should be obtained. Similarly, the student of clinical methods should obtain the patient's consent to proceed with the interview. For example:

> **Student:** Good morning, Mr. Cummings. My name is Bill Sams, and I am a student doctor learning how to interview patients. Your doctor gave me your name. Would you be willing to talk to me for a few minutes?

The interview can proceed as planned after the patient gives verbal permission. In the unlikely event that the patient does not want to be interviewed, the student should politely thank the patient and leave the room. Even when patients have previously given their permission for a student interview, some change their minds. Students should respect these wishes and not pressure such patients into agreeing to the interview.

ESTABLISHING INITIAL RAPPORT

Establishing rapport may be the most important part of the interview. The doctor-patient relationship begins at the moment the physician and the patient see each other, before any words are uttered. The patient and the physician will each make many judgments about the other before they establish verbal contact. Body posture, eye contact, interest level, and numerous other nonverbal cues will communicate important information to both the patient and the doctor. In general, the key to rapport is to demonstrate interest in the patient as a person. This can be demonstrated by showing concern and attention. Appearing hurried, bored, exhausted, or distracted can seriously undermine the relationship with the patient.

In addition to demonstrating interest, physicians should remember the following basic rule to help establish and maintain rapport:

Respond to patients' emotional reactions whenever they occur.

For example, if the patient shows some emotional reaction even as the physician first meets him or her, this can be acknowledged in the very beginning of the interview. If the patient is writhing in pain, the physician can acknowledge this before beginning an explanation about the purposes of the intended interview. Sometimes this acknowledgment can occur as part of the introduction itself. In a student interview, the student could say something like the following:

Student: Hello. I am John Downing, a student doctor. You seem to be in pain. Is there anything I can do for you?

Of course, there are numerous ways for physicians to respond appropriately to patients' emotions. Some of these modes have already been discussed in Chapter 3. Reflection is one of the most effective interventions. The student can comment on observed patient feelings, including pain, frustration, and sadness. These comments let patients know that their feelings have been noticed and that the feelings count for something. Such reflective comments usually help patients discuss their feelings and build doctor-patient rapport. The following are all examples of reflective comments that might be made in the very beginning of interviews:

Student: I see that you seem quite uncomfortable.
or
You appear to be in great pain.
or
I can tell that you seem a bit down.

When students or physicians make initial reflective comments about patients' emotions, especially early in the interview, some care must be taken to name feeling states that are relatively nonjudgmental and "near the surface." No depth interpretations should be made. Physicians should not begin interviews with heavily interpretive statements such as "You seem quite enraged" or "You are obviously despondent." Patients may experience such statements as intrusive, derogatory, or humiliating.

In practice, patients are forgiving of physicians who are genuinely trying to empathize with their distress, even if the physicians are slightly "off base" in their initial understanding. In such instances patients are quite willing to correct initial misunderstandings. For example, if the physician makes an incorrect statement about the patient's being distressed, the patient usually clarifies the situation:

Student: You seem to be in pain right now.

Patient: Actually, I'm mostly upset because I can't get my doctors to tell me what's the matter with me.

Student: I can understand why that might be disturbing. Would you be willing to tell me some more about that?

If the patient demonstrates an emotion and the student quite properly acknowledges the feeling, the student can continue reflecting and legitimating feelings, as described in Chapter 3, until the patient is ready to proceed with the rest of the interview.

Occasionally, a patient assigned to a student for a practice interview might complain directly about "being a guinea pig." Although this is unusual, students should be aware that this affective complaint does occur and should be responded to like any other demonstration of emotion. Because the student is the target of the emotion, the patient's affect may generate such anxiety in the student that it may be difficult to respond. Reflection and legitimation can also be useful in this instance:

Student: Do you mind if I ask you a few questions?

Patient: Another student? I've had so many people asking me questions, I don't know whether I'm coming or going.

Student: It sounds like you feel that you've been put through the mill. You may just not want to talk to another student.

Patient: That's right. I haven't had a chance to rest since I was admitted, with all the doctors and nurses coming in all the time.

Student: I can certainly understand how you might not want to talk to another student. If you'd rather I leave, that's perfectly all right.

Patient: No. That's all right. You can ask me some questions. What do you want to know?

Many such initially resistant patients will be quite interested and willing to proceed with the interview if their initial feelings are recognized and accepted. Those patients who continue to be reluctant to be interviewed must have their wishes respected.

ESTABLISHING PATIENT COMFORT

After the introduction, statement of purpose, acquisition of patient consent for the interview, and establishment of initial rapport, the student should establish patient comfort before beginning the rest of the interview. This intervention indicates the student's concern for the patient's comfort and indicates the student's willingness to help if possible. Establishing comfort is accomplished by a simple question such as the following:

> **Student:** Before I ask you about your illness itself, I want to check—how are you feeling right now?

This gives the patient the opportunity to tell the student how he or she is feeling at the moment. The response might be a physical or emotional answer, but the student has been given an important piece of information about the patient. If the patient is hot or cold, in pain, or thirsty, the student should ask whether he or she can do anything to help. If the patient responds with an emotional response such as "I am scared that I have cancer," the student can proceed with relationship skills to help the patient express and cope with these feelings (see Chapter 3).

In summary, the opening to the medical interview has five important components. There are many ways to open medical interviews, but the structure reviewed in this chapter represents one effective approach. The separate steps are summarized below.

Steps for an Effective Opening

Introduction	Hello, I am John Smith, a student doctor. Dr. Jones gave me your name.
Establish goals	Dr. Jones suggested that I talk with you about your illness to help me learn how to interview patients.
Obtain patient consent	Is that OK with you?
Establish initial rapport	You seem to be in pain.
Establish patient comfort	How are you feeling right now?

REFERENCES

1. Lipkin M Jr, Frankel R, Beckman H, et al: Performing in the interview. In Lipkin M Jr, Putnam SM, Lazare A, editors: *The medical interview: clinical care, education, and research,* New York, 1995, Springer.

CHAPTER

8 Chief Complaint and Survey of Problems

After the introduction, the opening of the interview, and the development of initial rapport, the physician usually proceeds directly to the next two steps: the chief complaint and the survey of problems.

ELICITING THE CHIEF COMPLAINT

The chief complaint is the primary reason for the patient's seeking medical attention. By convention, this is stated in the patient's own words and usually recorded in the medical record in quotation marks. Most commonly, the physician asks a question something like the following:

Physician: What brought you here today?
or
How can I help you?
or
What is bothering you now?

Student physicians in an interviewing course will not be able to diagnose or treat a patient's problem, so a more appropriate question eliciting the chief complaint would be something like this:

Student: What problem brought you to the hospital (or clinic)?

The patient's answer will be recorded verbatim in the medical record as the patient's chief complaint. For example:

Patient: I couldn't catch my breath.

Occasionally patients will answer this question with a medical diagnosis rather than a description of symptoms. For example, a patient might respond in the following manner:

Patient: It was my emphysema.
or
They told me it was an embolus.

If patients provide a diagnosis rather than a symptom, they can be asked to describe exactly what they experienced themselves that made them seek medical attention. For example:

Student: I understand that you were told that you had an embolus, but I would like to know exactly what you experienced that led you to come to the doctor.

In response to this type of direct question, patients will usually be able to provide a statement concerning the symptoms that they experienced. For example:

Patient: Oh, I got really short of breath.

RESPONDING TO EMOTIONS

Occasionally patients will provide information in a chief complaint that is highly charged with emotion. When this occurs, it is usually best to respond to this emotion when it first becomes apparent. For example, a patient might say something such as the following:

Patient: I was so short of breath I thought I was dying.

When this degree of emotional intensity accompanies a report of symptoms, the student can respond effectively by using any one of many different interventions. However, brief reflective comments can be appropriate and supportive. For example:

Student: I am sure that must have been very frightening.

This type of comment usually invites the patient to discuss his or her feelings in more detail. For example:

Patient: I've never been so scared. I just couldn't get my breath. It was terrible.

After a patient acknowledges and discusses some significant feelings, the student can indicate his or her acceptance of these feelings in many ways. One effective technique is the use of direct, validating (or legitimating) comments. For example:

Student: I can certainly understand your fear. I would have felt the same way myself.

INITIAL FACILITATION

The use of facilitating comments is an open-ended method of encouraging a patient to keep talking without interfering or influencing the direction of the patient's comments. Facilitation can be verbal or nonverbal. Examples of minimal and nonintrusive facilitation include head nodding or saying "uh-huh" or "yes" in response to a patient's comments. Such interventions, although minimal, let the patient know that the interviewer is listening and encourage the patient to keep talking.

Use more specific facilitations to directly ask the patient to continue:

Physician: Please tell me more.
or
Please go on.

When a patient rambles or discusses many different themes together in a disjointed manner, the physician can help guide the interview in a more efficient way by using facilitation to direct the patient:

Physician: Before you tell me about the headache, can we first concentrate on the chest pain? Please tell me a bit more about the chest pains you've been having.

The patient will usually respond to such open-ended facilitation by discussing the points that are most important to him or her as a patient. This provides the physician with crucial information that could not be obtained as easily by more closed-ended questions that focus on the physician's concerns. The patient will generally respond in his or her own words about the symptoms of the chest pain that were most troubling. The psychosocial context might also emerge. For example, the patient might say something like the following:

Patient: Well, last Sunday I was almost finished mowing the lawn when I suddenly got short of breath and I noticed a heavy, tight feeling in my chest.

Continued facilitation is still appropriate if the patient is talking about relevant symptoms. Thoughtful and attentive silence can also serve as a potent facilitator. If this is uncomfortable or feels socially inappropriate, the interviewer can provide a more direct facilitative comment:

> **Physician:** Could you tell me some more about the heavy, tight feeling?

This type of facilitation will usually encourage the patient to talk more about the symptoms of interest.

> **Patient:** Well, I've never really had anything like it before. It hurt, but it was more like an ache than a sharp pain. I thought it might be gas, but I couldn't get it to go away. And then I noticed that the tight feeling spread to my back and down my left arm.

CHECKING

Checking is a key and underused assessment skill.

Checking is the physician's attempt to summarize the information that he or she has just received from the patient. This single intervention is one of the most important data-gathering skills for several reasons. It is the only way for the physician to check the accuracy of what he or she thinks the patient has just said. Interviewers may at times misunderstand the meaning of what the patient has said or even specific data that patients have given them. Checking allows the physician a chance to correct any misunderstandings. Checking also communicates a sense to the patient that the physician is listening and trying to understand. Such efforts usually contribute to overall rapport.

In addition to other uses, checking provides a therapeutic "breathing space." When a lull occurs in the interview or the physician needs to make a decision about which direction to proceed, checking can be used to review what has already been covered. The physician can use these pauses to gracefully consider alternative strategies for the rest of the interview. The nature of the patient's response to the checking may itself help the physician decide on the course of the rest of the interview. The physician may use checking in the following manner:

> **Physician:** Let me take a moment to make sure that I've understood you correctly. You said that you were just finishing mowing the lawn last Sunday when you noticed the sudden onset of a sharp pain in your chest and had trouble breathing.

SURVEY OF PROBLEMS

The survey of problems is an extremely important part of the interview and, like checking, is often overlooked. A skillful survey of problems can dramatically increase the efficiency of the interviewing process. In the survey of problems the physician attempts to briefly scan the full range of a patient's problems. To begin the survey, the physician asks the following key question:

Physician: What else is bothering you?
or simply
What else?

Completing the survey of problems in the early stages of the interview is important because otherwise physicians sometimes lose valuable time by focusing on problems that are not the most clinically significant or the most distressing to patients. The survey usually does not take long, and it allows the physician to determine the full range of the patient's problems. After the physician (1) elicits the chief complaint, (2) responds to the initial emotions, (3) facilitates the open-ended expression of more details about the chief complaint, and (4) checks what he or she has heard, the physician should proceed with the survey of problems.

Physician: Now that you have told me what problem brought you to the hospital initially, I want to ask you about your other problems. I will come back to the chest pain in a few moments. What other problems do you have?
Patient: Well, I have had some prostate trouble.

As with the original chief complaint, the physician should follow this new complaint with open-ended facilitative interventions to collect more details about the problem, respond to emotions that are connected with this problem, and check the information obtained after several comments have been made by the patient.

Physician: Can you tell me some more about the prostate problem?
Patient: Well, I dribble, and it takes a long time to finish. I'm afraid I might need an operation.
Physician: So, in addition to this chest pain you have a problem with urinating. You take a long time to pass your water, and there is some dribbling. You're also concerned that you might need an operation. What other problems do you have?
Patient: I also have trouble with migraine headaches.
Physician: Can you say more about the headaches?
Patient: I have had them all my life. Sometimes they are so bad I can't

stand it and I have to miss work and go to the emergency room for a shot. I haven't had one in three months now.

Physician: So, you have this chest pain, prostate trouble, and migraine headaches. I want to hear more about each of these problems. But now I still want you to tell me what other problems you have.

Many patients are reluctant to tell physicians about some problems that are particularly sensitive. Sometimes patients are so anxious about these problems that they postpone discussing them to the end of the interview, when the physician may not be willing or able to spend more time. The source of the patient's anxiety may be an overwhelming health concern such as the fear of cancer. For example, the patient in the preceding dialogue might be afraid that the stomach pain he has been experiencing is cancer. If the fear of cancer is strong, he might avoid bringing the pain up at all because of anxiety. At the end of the interview the anxiety of not discussing the abdominal pain might be stronger than the anxiety of discussing it. This can lead to an unpleasant tension when the physician is about to leave the room, as the patient awkwardly says something like the following:

Patient: Doctor, could I ask you something else? I've been having this stomach pain.

This type of interaction can be troubling for both patients and physicians. It can lead to tension in the relationship. More important, the physician may simply not have the time at the end of the interview to deal with this new problem adequately. The new problem may be quite important; sometimes it is the patient's hidden or unconscious chief complaint. In addition to the type of problem mentioned in the dialogue, patients usually leave sexual, psychiatric, or interpersonal problems to the end of the interview, either because of the anxiety they arouse or because patients fear that the physician may not consider these problems important or "medical." Studies indicate that these "end of the interview" or "Oh, by the way, doctor ..." statements occur in up to 20% of interviews.[1] Permitting this covert complaint to remain uncovered until the end of the interview usually leads to inadequate care and certainly to inefficient care. A proper survey of problems can often eliminate this difficulty.

PROBING TO COMPLETENESS

The survey of problems is not complete until the physician has probed to completeness. The interviewer should continue asking, "What else?" until the patient convincingly indicates that all the problems have been mentioned. It is important for the physician to indicate that he or she is not rushed in this task and sincerely wants to hear at least briefly about all of the patient's problems. The physician must give the patient full attention and watch closely for nonverbal messages from the patient about uncomfortable topics. If the patient demonstrates ambivalence about talking about some problems, the physician should do what he or she can to encourage the patient to talk about these more anxiety-provoking problems. For example:

> **Patient:** Well, now that you mention it, there is something else that has been on my mind . . . (pause)
> **Physician:** Yes . . . I would like to hear more about it.

The physician should continue this type of interested inquiry until the patient clearly indicates that all problems have been mentioned.

Some physicians may wonder why it is so important to elicit all the patient's problems. Some physicians may believe that sexual, psychiatric, and interpersonal problems may be beyond the scope of the physician to manage. The information necessary for the physician to understand these problems may take a great deal of time to elaborate. While these are all understandable concerns, students must realize that a patient's sexual, psychiatric, and interpersonal problems belong in the interview: they have a direct effect on the course and outcome of a patient's illness, on health care use, on the patient's coping with illness, on the quality of life, and on overall life adjustment.[2]

Physicians do not need to be experts on all these sensitive issues to take some history about them. If there is not time in one interview to address all the concerns that arise out of a thorough survey of problems, some of the topics can be postponed to another interview. It is still important and efficient in the long run to take a complete survey of problems for every new patient seen and to survey the patient at least briefly during follow-up visits.

Some patients with significant psychiatric and psychosocial problems bring up problems such as impotence, family conflict, fears of dying, and work problems, in addition to problems such as chest pain, migraine headaches, and prostate trouble. The physician can decide which problems to investigate and in which order of priority they can reasonably be investigated. Some problems may need to be referred tc outside experts or agencies.

NEGOTIATING PRIORITIES

Once the complete problem list has been developed through a systematic survey of problems, the physician should negotiate the priority of investigation with the patient.[2] This should be a collaborative effort guided by the physician's medical understanding of which problems might be most imminently threatening to the patient's health and balanced by the patient's personal hierarchy of concerns. When there is conflict between the doctor's and the patient's list of priorities, the order in which problems will be addressed should be directly negotiated. In general, the physician should let the patient determine the order of priority as much as possible. For example:

Physician: Now that we have outlined all of your problems, I'd like to hear from you about which ones bother you most.

Patient: I'd really like to know more about this prostate thing. I think that's what is causing my problem with sex.

Physician: I'm also concerned about your prostate and I see it's a problem for you. I'll make sure that we get to it, but if it's acceptable to you, I think we need to make sure that we've dealt appropriately with the chest pain. There may be something we need to take care of right away.

Patient: OK.

PATIENT EXPECTATIONS

Sometimes the patient's expectations of the physician are quite clear. In other cases, however, the patient's expectations are less clear. Even if they are not immediately clear, the specific desires of the patient are much more important in cases in which the patient has a chronic illness with difficulty adapting or some other psychosocial problem.

For example, a patient who is impotent because of diabetes may only want to talk about how the impotence is affecting his marital relationship. To bring back his sexual abilities, the patient may simply want a pill or he may be interested in a penile implant. Asking directly about the patient's expectations can increase rapport in the relationship, improve efficiency in the interview, and achieve a more satisfied patient in the long run.[3] If the physician knows what the patient wants, the physician will have an easier time satisfying the patient.

Patient expectations can be elicited directly:

Physician: Please tell me as specifically as you can how you think I might be able to help you with your problem with sex.

PATIENT'S IDEAS ABOUT THE MEANING OF THE ILLNESS

At times the patient's ideas about the meaning of the illness are quite clear. This may not always be the case. For example, the patient with some rather obscure abdominal pain might be concerned that cancer could be causing the pain. Alternatively, the concern might be social embarrassment from the passing of flatus. Unless the physician knows the patient's ideas about the meaning of the symptom (i.e., the patient's "explanatory model"), the physician will be inefficient in his or her care and may not be able to meet the patient's needs.[4]

The physician should directly ask the patient what he or she thinks could be causing the symptom. For example:

> **Physician:** Could you tell me what you think might be causing this stomach pain?
>
> **Patient:** I don't know, you're the doctor. That's why I came to you.
>
> **Physician:** Of course I am the doctor, and I will do what I can to help. But it will help me if you could tell me what thoughts have crossed your mind about what could be causing these problems.

Some patients may be unwilling to discuss their own ideas about the meaning of the illness, even with encouragement. However, when given an opportunity, many patients will be able to discuss their fears and ideas directly with the physician. This discussion can contribute to the efficiency of the doctor-patient interaction, as well as to the ability of the physician to reassure the patient. It can also enhance patient satisfaction. For example:

> **Patient:** Well, I know it's probably nothing. But my father died of colon cancer, and I'm kind of worried that I might have the same problem.
>
> **Physician:** I'm glad you could tell me that. It will help me understand your problem. After we talk about your pain and perhaps do some tests, I will do what I can to reassure you about your concern about cancer.

REFERENCES

1. White J, Levinson W, Roter D: "Oh, by the way"—the closing moments of the medical interview, *J Gen Intern Med* 9:24-28, 1994.
2. Cole S, Saravay S, Levinson R: The biopsychosocial model of illness. In Stoudemire A, editor: *An introduction to human behavior*, ed 3, Philadelphia, 1997, JB Lippincott.
3. Lazare A: The interview as a clinical negotiation. In Lipkin M Jr, Putnam SM, Lazare A, editors: *The medical interview: clinical care, education, and research*, New York, 1995, Springer.
4. Johnson TM, Hardt EJ, Kleinman A: Cultural factors in the medical interview. In Lipkin M Jr, Putnam SM, Lazare A, editors: *The medical interview: clinical care, education, and research*, New York, 1995, Springer.

CHAPTER

9 History of Present Illness (Problem Exploration)

The history of the present illness is an elaborated description of the patient's chief complaint and is the most important structural element of the medical history. Obtaining an accurate account of the patient's present illness in an efficient manner while also maintaining rapport is a key challenge of the medical interview.

Constructing the history of the present illness represents the physician's effort to understand the full story of the development and expression of the chief complaint in the context of the patient's life. The chief complaint could be a pain somewhere (e.g., chest pain), a symptom of discomfort (e.g., fatigue), a loss of usual function (e.g., inability to walk), or a troublesome body change (e.g., numbness in the fingertips). A psychiatric symptom such as depression or anxiety can also be the chief complaint.

The history of the present illness is different for every patient and provides essential information for optimal diagnosis and management. It also serves as a useful summary of the patient's problems for communication purposes with other caregivers.

NARRATIVE THREAD

The physician's goal in understanding the history of the present illness is to obtain a coherent, orderly portrait of the development of the patient's chief complaint. Lipkin[1] describes how the physician elicits the story of the patient's illness by developing a "narrative thread" linking the chronologic emergence of symptoms with the overall life circumstances of the patient. This requires considerably more skill than obtaining a recitation of relevant signs and symptoms; the physician must have the ability to understand the development and impact of an illness as one unified entity in the life of a unique patient. The physician cannot obtain this narrative thread from a patient as one can take a blood pressure. Rather, the physician must work in partnership with the patient to develop an accurate and useful understanding of the illness in the patient's life.

The distinction between a disease and an illness is useful at this point. As described by Kleinman et al,[2] "disease" refers to a physiologic, biologic disorder. Illness refers to a pattern of symptoms experienced by an individual: pain, discomfort, disability, and dysfunction. An individual may suffer from a disease (e.g., hypertension or occult cancer) without experiencing any illness. Similarly, a person may suffer from an illness (e.g., abdominal pain and disability) without any diagnosable disease. The narrative thread, therefore, refers primarily to the experience of the illness and not to the disease. Insofar as the patient may have already received objective confirmation (such as echocardiography) of an underlying disease related to his or her illness experience, these disease-related data also become embedded in the narrative thread of the history of the present illness.

To make the story coherent, the narrative thread must ascertain the natural lifetime sequence from the early stages of the interview:

> **Physician:** You mentioned that you noticed this sudden onset of chest pain just as you finished mowing the lawn on Sunday. Was this your very first episode of chest pain, or have you ever had chest pain before?

To continue the development of the narrative thread while retaining this focus on orderly chronology, the most important question is generally, "What happened next?"

> **Physician:** After you first noticed the pain on Sunday, what happened next?
>
> **Patient:** I went inside to tell my wife.
>
> **Physician:** After you went inside to tell your wife, what happened next?

The physician may find it necessary to interrupt the patient's narrative to ask some clarifying questions. After the patient provides this clarification, the physician should generally return to the question, "What next?" in order to continue the narrative thread.

> **Patient:** My wife said she was taking me to the hospital.
>
> **Physician:** Before we go further, can you describe the pain in some more detail?
>
> **Patient:** It kind of grabbed me—deep down, tight.
>
> **Physician:** Can you show me exactly where it hurt?
>
> **Patient:** Right here in my chest, and then it went down my left arm and into my back.

Physician: How bad was it?
Patient: Not too bad at first, but then I had trouble catching my breath.
Physician: Did you notice anything else unusual?
Patient: No, that was about all I noticed that I can remember.
Physician: OK, so you noticed a dull, tight, hard pain in your chest that went down your arm. It wasn't too bad at first, but then it started to bother you a whole lot when you got short of breath.
Patient: That's right.
Physician: What happened next?

In terms of question format, the skilled interviewer generally starts with open-ended questions to establish the broad outlines of the story. As the patient recounts symptoms and patterns, the interviewer becomes more focused and uses progressively more specific and narrow questions to fill in specific details. Eventually, final details must be elicited by using closed questions. This progressive narrowing of focus has been called an "open-to-closed-cone" style of questioning.[3]

The overall process of developing the present illness as a narrative thread establishes coherence and an order that helps make sense of the patient's experience, both to the doctor and to the patient. For the patient, it may represent the first time that he or she has actually articulated the pattern of symptom development in this logical manner. An orderly recounting of symptoms and the sense that the doctor understands this can be quite reassuring.

SEVEN CONTENT ITEMS

The seven core dimensions of any complaint must be investigated in detail.[4] In general, these seven content areas provide information necessary for the physician to recognize patterns of illness and to generate diagnostic hypotheses. A common challenge for the interviewer in investigating each of these areas is to obtain specific information without prematurely closing off the open-ended phase of the interview.

In general, each of the seven content areas is investigated in detail after the open-ended phase of the interview. In reality, few interviews proceed in this linear fashion and follow an idealized open-to-closed cone. In practice, even skilled interviewers usually interrupt or direct a patient in the early stages of an interview to prevent the physician from getting "lost" in a sea of seemingly unrelated details. When it is necessary, the physician can interrupt briefly to gather needed details by using closed questions and then return to an open-ended format. Care and discretion must be used to prevent such an interruption from terminating the open-ended portion of the interview.

Location

The physician must have a precise understanding of the location of the problem. At times the patient may speak in generalities or use a vocabulary that is not familiar to the physician. When this occurs, the physician must ask the patient to clarify the words. For example, a patient may indicate that his or her stomach hurts. It is sometimes useful to ask the patient to show the doctor specifically where it hurts. If the open-ended portion of the history was interrupted, the patient can be redirected in a more open-ended manner after a specific detail has been clarified.

Physician: Can you take one finger and show me exactly where it hurts? (clarifying question)
Patient: Right here, doctor. (patient points to the location)
Physician: OK. Can you now describe the pain to me in more detail? (return to more open-ended questioning)

Quality

It is important for the patient to attempt to describe the quality of the symptom, because different disease syndromes can produce specific recognizable patterns of complaints. For example, a pain may be stabbing, sharp, dull, throbbing, or continuous.

It is usually best for the doctor to ask this question in as open-ended a way as possible.

Physician: Could you describe the pain? What is it like?

Patients usually know what the doctor wants in asking for such a description. However, if the patient seems to be at a loss for words, the physician can provide some useful guidance:

Patient: What do you mean "describe the pain"? Doctor, it just hurt.
Physician: OK, I guess I mean I would like to hear a little bit more about what it actually felt like. Was it sharp or dull? Did it come and go or just stay there all the time?

Severity

It is important for the physician to get some ideas about how severe the discomfort, sensation, or pain was or is to the patient. This can sometimes be ascertained by noting nonverbal signals of acute discomfort by the patient, but the question about severity should also be asked directly.

Physician: How bad was the pain?
Patient: It was terrible.
Physician: Was it the worst pain you've ever experienced?
Patient: No, my kidney stone was actually worse.

A crude analogue scale can be very useful in measuring subjective levels of discomfort.

Physician: Could you tell me how bad this headache pain has been?
Patient: Well, it's sort of achy and pressured.
Physician: Well, on a scale of one to ten, where one represents no pain and ten represents the worst pain you've ever experienced, how bad was your last headache?
Patient: I guess about a five or a six.

Timing

As described previously, the timing of the symptoms and associated responses is essential to the development of a coherent narrative thread. The physician needs to know when each symptom or problem began and also needs to know the rough chronology of the development of the problem. The physician occasionally needs to briefly interrupt the patient's story to make sure the timing of events is clear. If the patient begins reciting an array of symptoms without providing the details of the timing, it is helpful to interrupt:

Physician: So what is it that brought you to the clinic today? (open-ended elicitation of the chief complaint)
Patient: It's these headaches. They're getting worse and worse. Now I've started to become nauseated, and I threw up yesterday.
Physician: Can you say some more about the headaches?
Patient: Well, yesterday was just terrible. The pain started slowly just as I woke up, and it got worse and worse during the day. I had to leave work, and that's when I went home and threw up. I took some of my wife's pain medicine and was able to go to sleep.
Physician: What medicine was that? (interrupts for clarification)
Patient: I think it was Tylenol Number Three.
Physician: And can you tell me when this problem first started? (physician interrupts to establish the time frame)
Patient: I guess I had my first bad headache like this about two years ago.

Physician: OK, so can you tell me some more about what it was like when the headaches started about two years ago? (physician returns to more open-ended questioning)

As new or associated symptoms develop that are related to the problem being discussed, the physician needs to know about the timing of these related symptoms:

Patient: Then I began throwing up with the headaches.
Physician: About when did you begin to throw up with the headache?
Patient: I guess the first time I began to throw up was about six weeks ago.

Context

The context of the symptom development is essential to an understandable narrative thread and can give many clues for diagnosis and management:

Physician: Can you tell me where you are or what you are doing when you tend to get these headaches?
Patient: I guess they mostly start at work.
Physician: Can you say some more about that?
Patient: I guess they mostly come in the afternoons, especially on days that are very busy and when I feel pressured.
Physician: Is there anything else that comes to mind about the situations in which these headaches seem to develop?
Patient: Not really.

Modifying Factors

The physician needs to find out what the patient has done to try to help himself or herself feel better and what types of things may make the symptoms worse:

Physician: Could you tell me what tends to help this pain?
Patient: Well, if I lie down in a dark, quiet room, the pain calms down a little.
Physician: Have you tried any medicines?
Patient: Aspirin or Tylenol used to help, but they don't work anymore. Yesterday I took that Tylenol Number Three. Sometimes I need to go to an emergency room for a shot to stop the pain.
Physician: What kinds of things make the headaches worse?
Patient: If I cough, it hurts. Looking at bright light hurts. Trying to concentrate hurts. That's about it.

Associated Signs and Symptoms

The physician should inquire about associated signs and symptoms. These can provide essential additional information for diagnosis or management of a patient's problem.

Physician: When you get these headaches, what other sensations or feelings do you get?
Patient: Well, sometimes I get nauseated. I feel weak and dizzy. If I try to walk, I feel unsteady on my feet.
Physician: Any other symptoms you can think of?
Patient: No.

Under the category of associated signs and symptoms, physicians ask patients directly about "pertinent positives and negatives." From their understanding of illness patterns, physicians inquire about specific symptoms and signs whose presence or absence can make a great deal of difference in clarifying the final diagnostic possibilities. However, beginning students will generally not know very much about what may or may not be "pertinent." This section of the interview will necessarily be much shorter for medical student interviews than for physician interviews.

COMPLETING THE NARRATIVE THREAD

As the patient provides responses to these seven content items, the physician should endeavor to weave the responses together into a coherent story within the patient's life experience. To accomplish this effectively often requires considerable skill. When the physician has completed the history of the present illness, he or she should have attained a good understanding of when the symptoms began; the quality, location, and severity of the symptoms; how the symptoms progressed; the timing of new symptoms; the context of the symptoms; modifying factors; and associated signs and symptoms.

COMPLETING THIS PROCESS FOR EVERY PROBLEM

The physician must obtain a history of the present illness for every current problem. If the patient has a problem with headaches, chest pain, back pain, and depression, each of these problems must be explored in the detail described previously. In practice, physicians may not have the time in the first meeting with a patient (particularly in an outpatient practice with patients having multiple nonacute problems) to obtain a complete history for every one of the problems. In this case, the physician and the patient should negotiate a priority problem list that can be addressed adequately in the time available. Other problems can usually wait for another appointment.

RESPONDING TO EMOTIONS THROUGHOUT

As patients recite the story of their illness, they will usually experience some emotional reactions. Physicians should always respond to these emotions.

Patients' emotions should never be ignored.

Each time a patient experiences an emotion that is overlooked by the physician, a wedge develops in the doctor-patient relationship and the physician has lost an opportunity for the development of deepened rapport.[5]

A sensitive physician can respond to a patient's emotions in numerous ways. A nonverbal acknowledgment is often sufficient. For example, a patient who becomes tearful may respond to a soft touch on the arm or to the physician's moving his or her chair a little closer (for support) and talking in a softer voice.

A reflective verbal intervention is suggested for situations in which the physician is uncertain of how to proceed. For example:

Physician: I can see that this is hard to talk about.

If the patient becomes more emotional and more tearful, it is important to stop the general informational direction of the interview and continue exploring and supporting the patient's emotional responses. This can be accomplished by using more reflective comments, legitimation, support, partnership, and respect (see Chapter 3), as well as by other intuitive or higher-order skills of the physician (see Chapters 15 and 16).

Some interviewers may wonder whether devoting time to the emotional domain may interfere with the other task of collecting data. To the contrary, research indicates that attention to patients' emotional responses seems to facilitate the task of gathering information, perhaps by improving overall doctor-patient rapport.[6]

EVALUATING THE IMPACT OF THE ILLNESS ON THE PATIENT'S QUALITY OF LIFE

To understand a patient's illness and to facilitate coping, the physician evaluates the impact of the illness on the patient's quality of life. This information forms part of the present illness. The physician should explore the effect of the illness on the patient's general functioning. This includes the impact on (1) interpersonal relationships (especially spouse, significant other, and family), (2) work, (3) sexual relationships, and (4) emotional stability.

After the physician has developed the narrative thread, he or she will already have obtained a great deal of information about the effect of the illness on the patient's quality of life. This is especially true if the physician has responded to the emotions the patient has manifested. The physician should then complete the quality-of-life evaluation:

Physician: I'm interested in hearing more about how this illness has affected your life in general.
Patient: What do you mean?
Physician: I'd like to hear about the impact this illness has had on your life, your home situation, your work, and things like that.
Patient: OK. It's been hard. My work has fallen down because I've had to be out so much. I've been very tense, and I think I'm starting to take things out on my family.
Physician: Can you say some more about how this has affected your work?
Patient: I'm a data analyst for a large computer company. I have a lot of responsibility and a lot of deadlines to meet. I've been falling behind.
Physician: You said you've been tense and taking it out on your family. Can you say some more about that?
Patient: I'm worried and tense all the time. I yell at the kids a lot, and I can't really talk to my wife.
Physician: How has this affected your sex life?
Patient: Well, I've been out of sorts lately, and sex has been one of the first things to go.

Throughout the evaluation of the quality of life, the form of the questions can make a great difference in the patient's willingness to talk openly about psychosocial problems. This is especially true for topics like sexual adjustment, about which patients may be embarrassed or sensitive. For example, it is usually much more productive for the physician to ask *how* a symptom has affected someone's life rather than whether a symptom *has* had an effect. The following question may not be the most effective form:

Physician: Has this pain changed your sex life?
Patient: Not really.

In general, the following form of this question is usually more productive:

Physician: How has this pain affected your sex life?
Patient: Well, things have kind of slowed down a little.

Although this distinction is subtle, the style of questioning can make a definite difference in the way a patient responds to the physician's inquiries. When asked *how* a symptom has affected his or her life, a patient may feel encouraged to talk more openly, because the physician seems to expect a positive response and has given permission to talk about the problem. In contrast, when a physician asks whether or not a symptom *has* changed a patient's life, the patient may feel defensive and embarrassed to admit a problem. As students gain experience in eliciting this quality-of-life information, it becomes clear that different patients respond in different ways, even when suffering from similar illnesses. For example, some patients are most distressed by the loss of sleep, others by pain, and others by a change in sexual function. Family responses to illness are also quite different. When facing similar illness situations, one family might become more closely bonded and another might threaten to disintegrate.

Thus, by talking with patients about how a set of symptoms affects their quality of life, the physician attempts to develop a picture of the overall impact of the illness on general functioning and adaptation. This inquiry enables the physician to learn of the most distressing aspects of an illness for one specific patient and his or her family. By understanding the impact of the illness on the patient's quality of life, the physician can manage the patient better. Research indicates that physicians who inquire about the impact of symptoms are more likely to recognize emotional distress in their patients.[6] Treatment planning that takes quality-of-life issues into consideration is much more likely to be realistically accepted and followed by patients. Other interventions can be designed specifically to assist patient adaptation in the particular areas most problematic for patients.

REFERENCES

1. Lipkin M Jr: The medical interview and related skills. In Branch WT, editor: *The office practice of medicine*, ed 3, Philadelphia, 1994, WB Saunders.
2. Kleinman A, Eisenberg L, Good B: Culture, illness, and care: clinical lessons from anthropological and cross-cultural research, *Arch Intern Med* 88:251-258, 1978.
3. Goldberg D, Steele JJ, Smith C, et al: *Training family practice residents to recognize psychiatric disturbances*, Rockville, Md, 1983, National Institute of Mental Health.
4. Morgan WL, Engel GL: *The clinical approach to the patient*, Philadelphia, 1969, WB Saunders.
5. Suchman T, Beckman H, Frankel R: A model of empathic communication in the medical interview, *JAMA* 277:1680-1681, 1997.
6. Roter DL, Hall JA, Kern DE, et al: Improving physician's interviewing skills and reducing patients' emotional distress: a randomized clinical trial, *Arch Int Med* 155:1877-1884, 1995.
7. Hall JA, Roter DL, Katz NR: Meta-analysis of correlates of provider behavior in medical encounters, *Medical Care* 26:657-675, 1988.

CHAPTER

10 Medical History

The medical history is the record of the patient's past experiences with illnesses and medical treatments. Some of this information will already have been elicited in the elaboration of the history of the present illness. The ideal history of the present illness will include the elements of the medical history as well as family history, social history, and a review of systems that pertain to the patient's present complaints. (These other items will be discussed in the chapters that follow.) At times the systematic inquiry into medical history and other areas of the history will uncover additional information that applies to understanding the present illness better. When this occurs, the new information should be incorporated into the eventual write-up of the present illness.

The information in the medical history is important to collect in a thorough but efficient manner, because it often has great effect on eventual patient management. Most physicians develop a set of routine, relatively closed-ended questions for this part of the interview to ensure that all important areas of inquiry are covered systematically. When new problems are uncovered that need to be investigated, the style of questioning can change appropriately to a more open-ended form. In outpatient settings, because of time constraints and the lack of urgency of this information for immediate management, some physicians develop strategies for completing this database over several visits. However, whether this information is collected during the first visit or over several visits, it needs to be completed for every new patient.

The medical history comprises these content areas: (1) hospitalizations, (2) surgeries, (3) illnesses, (4) injuries, (5) medications, (6) allergies, (7) pregnancies (for women), (8) exposures, (9) health maintenance, and (10) psychiatric problems. Each of these general topics is discussed in this chapter with sample questions that might be useful.

It is usually helpful to introduce the medical history part of the interview by letting the patient know that the investigation of the current problem has been completed and that a different format and style of questioning will be used in conducting the evaluation of the medical history. This introduction can contribute to efficiency of interviewing by letting the patient know the kind of information that is desired. For example:

Physician: I think I have a good understanding now of your problem with chest pain. I'd like to go on and ask a series of questions about other medical problems you may have had in the past.
Patient: OK.

HOSPITALIZATIONS

A relatively closed-ended question is usually sufficient to inquire about past hospitalizations and surgeries. For example:

Physician: Please tell me about your previous hospitalizations.

Some patients may become overly concerned about recounting exact details of previous hospitalizations, such as exact dates or exact symptoms. Similarly, some patients may think that the physician wants to hear the details of the symptoms that led to previous hospitalizations in the same way that the details of the present illness were discussed. Such patients need to be gently directed toward the kind of answers that are most appropriate for this phase of the interview. Consider the following example:

Physician: Please tell me about your previous hospitalizations.
Patient: Well, let's see. I had this stomach problem a while back. I think it was ten years ago . . . no, it may have been eleven . . . no. It was ten. They eventually decided it was a gallbladder problem. The pain was terrible, but it came and went. It took them a long time to figure things out, but they eventually decided to take out the gallbladder, and the pain went away. It started with a sharp pain right here, and then it went around . . .
Physician: Excuse me a moment, I'm sorry to interrupt. I appreciate your efforts to be very specific. But since we are a little short of time, I want to make sure you know that I only need a very rough idea of each time you have been in a hospital before and for what problem. For example, for your gallbladder operation, I only need to know about when it was taken out. I don't really need to know the symptoms that led up to the operation, and whether it was ten or eleven years ago is not really that important for what we need to accomplish now.

SURGERIES

Many significant surgeries will already have been mentioned in the patient's review of hospitalizations. However, since more and more surgery is now being performed on an outpatient basis, it is important to ask about surgeries as a separate category to make sure the area has been completely covered:

Physician: Besides the operations you've already mentioned, have you had any other surgeries?

ILLNESSES

The physician can investigate previous illnesses by using the same strategies discussed above. For example:

Physician: Now that we have discussed hospitalizations, can you tell me about any serious or troubling illnesses you have had in the past?

As the patient brings up past experiences with illness, the physician should find out general information concerning the severity of the illness, treatment, and outcome.

After the patient recounts his or her past illnesses, most physicians then mention other significant illnesses to try to make sure no other important past illnesses have been omitted:

Physician: Now I am going to mention a series of other common illnesses, and I would like to know if you have ever had one of them. Has anyone ever told you that you have high blood pressure? Heart disease? Kidney disease, stones, or bladder infections? Stomach problems or ulcers? Liver or gallbladder problems? Lung or breathing problems? Venereal disease (gonorrhea, syphilis, herpes, AIDS)? Arthritis? Anemia or problems with bleeding? Cancer? Diabetes? Thyroid problems? Nervous or emotional problems?

Beginning medical students usually need to make a list of these illnesses for reference as they talk to patients to make sure that the complete list is covered.

INJURIES

Physician: Have you ever had any serious accidents or injuries? (What happened? Did you break any bones? Were you hospitalized?)

MEDICATIONS

A complete and systematic review of the patient's experience with medications is essential. This must include over-the-counter medicines as well.

Physician: What medicines are you taking now? (What strength? How often do you take it? How often do you miss a dose?)
Physician: Are you taking any over-the-counter medications? Anything for sleep or bowels? Vitamins or pain pills?

The patient's past experience with medications is also essential.

Physician: What medications have you taken in the past?

ALLERGIES

Because patients may not remember to inform the physicians of allergies, this information must be elicited directly.

Physician: Do you have any allergies? (What kind of allergic reactions have you had? Have you had any allergic reaction to penicillin or injections used for x-ray studies?)

PREGNANCIES

Physician: Have you ever been pregnant? (How many times? Any problems or complications?)

EXPOSURES

Physician: In your work or other activities, have you been exposed to chemicals, dusts, or fumes that might be dangerous? (Are your work conditions safe? Are you exposed to any other dangerous situations that you are aware of?)

HEALTH MAINTENANCE

This section of the interview has alternately been called the health risk profile, health promotion, or preventive health care aspect of the history. Some traditional interviewing approaches do not include this information, but the trend in medicine has been to focus on these issues more and more. The questions below have been modeled after the contribution of Billings and Stoeckle,[1] who indicate that five general topics should be addressed.

The first topic is periodic health examinations:

> **Physician:** Do you have a regular doctor? How often do you get regular check-ups? When was your last dental exam? When did you last get your eyes checked? Do you check your breasts for lumps? Have you ever gotten a mammogram? When was your last Pap smear? Have you had your cholesterol measured?

The second topic area is immunizations:

> **Physician:** Did you get immunizations as a child? Which ones? Were you checked for German measles during pregnancy? Do you get annual flu shots (for the elderly or other patients at risk)?

The third topic area is injury prevention:

> **Physician:** How often do you use seat belts? Do you have smoke detectors? Tell me how to help prevent children from poisoning themselves (for parents). Have you checked your hot water temperatures (to prevent burns in children)? Has your home been checked for hazards (for the elderly)?

The fourth topic area is exercise:

> **Physician:** What do you do for exercise?

The fifth topic area is contraception and the prevention of sexually transmitted diseases:

> **Physician:** How often do you have sexual relations with another person? How often do you use birth control? What methods do you use? What concerns do you have about sexually transmitted diseases like AIDS? What precautions are you taking?

PSYCHIATRIC PROBLEMS

Many physicians quite properly elicit psychiatric history throughout the rest of the medical history. Previous psychiatric hospitalizations, illnesses, or medications can easily be investigated as part of this general topic. Because some patients and physicians do not routinely inquire into psychiatric problems, some screening time should be devoted to making sure that past psychiatric problems have not been omitted.

Physical problems that result from psychiatric problems (e.g., chest pain secondary to panic disorder or fatigue secondary to depression) are common in general medical practice.[2] In addition, psychiatric conditions that coexist with general medical problems contribute to excess morbidity, mortality, and the use of health services.[3] Physicians who tend to focus only on differential diagnoses of the physical symptoms often miss these conditions. By asking directly about past psychiatric history, physicians can often pick up psychiatric distress that contributes to impaired current functioning.

A review of the patient's psychiatric history can be accomplished quickly with the following type of questions:

Physician: What nervous or mental problems have you had? Have you ever had medication for your nerves? Have you ever been in counseling?

REFERENCES

1. Billings JA, Stoeckle JD: *The clinical encounter: a guide to the medical interview and case presentation*, ed 2, St Louis, 1998, Mosby.
2. Kroenke K, Spitzer RL, Williams JBW, et al: Physical symptoms in primary care: predictor of psychiatric disorders and functional impairment, *Arch Fam Med* 3:774-779, 1994.
3. Cole S, Saravay S: The biopsychosocial model of illness. In Stoudemire A, editor: *An introduction to human behavior*, ed 3, Philadelphia, 1997, JB Lippincott.

CHAPTER 11 Family History

The family history focuses on the health problems of the patient's closest relatives. This information can be especially important in investigating the possibility or implications of genetically transmitted diseases.

As the physician inquires about family illnesses, many of the patient's concerns about his or her own condition may emerge. The patient may also experience significant emotional reactions when discussing family illnesses. In both of these cases the physician should notice these concerns and reactions and respond to them. For example:

Physician: I'd like to ask a few questions about illnesses in your family. Please tell me about your parents' health.

Patient: My mother has high blood pressure, and my father is dead. He died of a heart attack five years ago.

Physician: I'm sorry. How old was he at the time?

Patient: Fifty-eight. My grandfather also died of a heart attack.

Physician: How old was your grandfather when he died?

Patient: I don't know for sure. Probably about sixty-five or so. Do you think I have heart disease too?

Physician: I can see why you might be concerned about your chest pains with this family history. I don't know yet whether there is a problem there or not. We still need to do the physical examination and a few tests. If you do have a heart problem, I want you to know there's a lot we can do for you to help prevent any major problems. We'll discuss our options in detail if we need to do anything.

The physician needs to inquire in detail about health problems and treatment of all first-degree relatives (parents, siblings, and children). When looking for general health problems that might "run" in a large family, the physician can use more open-ended global questions:

Physician: Are there any other illnesses that run in your family, in your cousins or aunts and uncles?

After specific information has been elicited, the physician will usually also ask whether anyone else in the family has ever had problems similar to the ones the patient is currently experiencing:

Physician: Has anyone else in the family ever had problems like yours?

When completing the family history, the physician will usually ask a few brief screening questions, mentioning the same illnesses surveyed at the end of the evaluation of the medical history (see Chapter 10).

Physician: Has anyone else in the family ever had trouble with high blood pressure? Kidneys or bladder? Lungs?

CHAPTER

12 Patient Profile and Social History

The patient profile and social history are important parts of the database. The information elicited in this part of the interview helps with both diagnosis and treatment planning. For example, a patient's life-style, family and cultural history, social environment, and employment situation significantly influence the expression of symptoms, decisions to seek treatment, levels of functional disability, and willingness to adhere to treatment strategies.

Similarly, family structure profoundly influences patient care and outcome. For example, cohesive families help patients cope and adapt to functional limitations. Alternatively, significant family conflict may be predictive of problematic outcome in a physical illness. Family stability is furthermore associated with adherence to medical regimens. Unfortunately, because the psychosocial aspects of a patient's life are so complex, students often have difficulty deciding how much of this information to pursue. Hours could be spent on this part of the interview alone. Students may be reassured to realize that this is also a significant challenge for experienced physicians.

There is often a difference between what experts recommend and what many physicians actually do. Medical textbooks routinely propose an extensive list of psychosocial areas that should be addressed (e.g., sibling relationships, developmental milestones, early work experiences, and relationships to parents when growing up).[1] In practice, however, most medical charts do not mention these topics,[2] and most physicians find it impractical to address all these topics with all patients.

Clinical discretion plays a key role in the determination of the balance between psychosocial exploration and more routine biologic evaluation. Different patients and different medical problems clearly influence the pattern and balance of questioning. When psychosocial variables seem to play a significant role in the etiology, exacerbation, or treatment of a medical problem, extensive evaluation of the social history becomes more critical.

This chapter reviews what can be considered the basic but adequate evaluation of the patient profile and social history. More extensive investigation is necessary for more complex cases. It is also worth noting that the evaluation of the social history is often different for inpatient and outpatient settings. For outpatients, physicians often use several visits to develop an adequate understanding of the patient profile and social history.

The basic patient profile and social history comprise the following components: (1) patient profile, (2) life-style risk factors, (3) stresses, and (4) support. Each of these dimensions will be considered separately.

PATIENT PROFILE

The patient profile represents the physician's understanding of a patient's uniqueness as a person. This generally includes three domains:

1. **Interpersonal relationships:** Ask about the patient's primary social (e.g., married, single, divorced, children, extended family, and friends) and sexual (activity, sexual orientation, and use of protection) relationships.
2. **Leisure activities:** Evaluate how the patient spends his or her time (e.g., work, daily activities, leisure, and organized groups).
3. **Other factors:** Note other factors the patient considers important to mention. Many physicians obtain some of this information at the beginning of an interview, while others elicit it throughout the interview or wait to investigate social history in detail after the physical evaluation is complete.

Regardless of when the physician chooses to evaluate the patient profile, he or she can introduce the topic by saying something like the following:

> **Physician:** Can you tell me a little about yourself as a person? I'd like to know a little about your family and the people who are important to you.

This type of open-ended question usually elicits a great deal of information about a patient's family and social relationships. The physician can follow the patient's leads as appropriate.

Given the prevalence of human immunodeficiency virus (HIV) and acquired immunodeficiency syndrome (AIDS) and the epidemic of other sexually transmitted diseases, the physician's inquiry into patterns of sexual behavior has become a requisite part of the general medical evaluation. Although many medical students and practicing physicians may be uncomfortable with this line of questioning, three basic questions should be incorporated into every complete medical history. An orienting statement can be helpful, before asking the three questions about sexual activity, orientation, and protection. For example:

> **Physician:** I now need to ask you some questions about your sexual life. I ask these questions of all my patients. Are you currently sexually active? Are you active with men, with women, or with both? Do you ever have unprotected sexual relations?

Because medical students and physicians find it so difficult to discuss sexual issues with their patients, Chapter 17 provides further guidance to this challenging topic.

After the physician learns something about the patient's social and sexual relationships, finding out more about how the patient spends his or her time (e.g., working, watching TV, keeping house, raising children, fishing, and going to church) is usually helpful.

> **Physician:** Can you tell me a little about how you spend your time?

The question about how a patient spends his or her time yields valuable information about the ability to function and cope with physical problems. It helps the physician learn about a patient's ability to work and function in the home with an illness. The question about time also yields information about the use of leisure time and activities such as church attendance that may be central to the lives of some patients.

After the physician has elicited information about social relationships and time, it is usually helpful to ask the patient at least one more open-ended question about himself or herself:

> **Physician:** What else would you like to tell me about yourself that you think might help me understand you better?

An open-ended question like this prompts the patient to select aspects of his or her life that may be central to future patient management.

HIGH-RISK HEALTH BEHAVIORS

Negative health habits are important risk factors for the development of future illnesses and need to be evaluated. Patients need to be asked about their smoking habits and their use of alcohol and nonprescription drugs. These include over-the-counter medicines, as well as substances of abuse (e.g., street drugs).

Since alcoholism is so common (about 20% of men have clinically significant alcoholism at some time in their lives) and since denial is so common among alcoholics, special interviewing techniques are usually required to elicit a history of alcoholism.[3] Most patients who have problems with alcohol do not openly admit to this difficulty, and when asked to specify amounts of alcohol consumed they will tend to minimize the amount.

The "CAGE" interview, which inquires about the effects of drinking rather than drinking itself, can be helpful in eliciting information suggestive of alcohol abuse.[4] The four letters in CAGE are used as a mnemonic device to remember the four important questions that should be asked of all patients to explore the possibility of alcohol abuse.

C Have you ever felt the need to **cut** down on your drinking?
A Do you ever get **annoyed** when people tell you to cut down on your drinking?
G Do you ever feel **guilty** about drinking too much?
E Have you ever needed an **"eye-opener"** in the mornings?

If the patient answers "yes" to any of the four questions of the CAGE model, the possibility of alcohol abuse is present and must be explored in much more detail. Interviewing patients about their drinking behavior is complex and difficult.[5] Physicians should also try to obtain an approximate amount of alcohol consumed, while realizing that the amount admitted to is almost always far less than the amount actually consumed. For example:

Physician: You say that you drink a beer or two each night. Are there any nights when you drink two or three six-packs?

When extremes of possible consumption are mentioned, patients are sometimes more willing to admit to heavier patterns of use.

Patients should also be asked about their use of illicit drugs. Some physicians ask these questions after they have inquired about prescription and nonprescription drugs. For example:

Physician: You've mentioned some medications prescribed by the doctor and some you've bought in drug stores. Have you ever used drugs for recreation? Have you ever used uppers or downers? Have you ever tried cocaine?

Physicians also need to inquire about smoking. For example:

Physician: Do you smoke? How much do you smoke? About how many packs do you smoke a day? For how many years have you smoked this much?

Total years of experience smoking are conventionally expressed in "pack-years." One year of smoking one pack of cigarettes a day equals one pack-year. Thus, 10 years of smoking three packs of cigarettes a day is counted as 30 pack-years.

HIGH-RISK LIFE SITUATION (HIGH STRESS AND LOW SUPPORT)

Social stress and social support are significant risk factors for most physical and psychiatric illnesses. For example, among patients experiencing their first heart attacks, those patients with low support and high stress were four times more likely to die of a repeat heart attack in the subsequent year.[6] This was true even after controlling for factors such as underlying cardiac condition, smoking and other negative health habits, visits to the doctor, and the prior state of health. The magnitude of this effect on outcome was as large as any physical risk factor (e.g., arrhythmias and congestive failure).

Because of the wealth of evidence that points to the important health consequences of life stress and social support, a brief consideration of both of these factors should be included in every new patient evaluation. This need not consume a great deal of time; two specific questions may be sufficient. However, more extensive evaluation may be necessary for patients who indicate problems in either of these areas.

Physician: Can you tell me a little about the kinds of stress you are under?

It is generally preferable to ask the question in the form listed above rather than asking the patient, "Are you under stress?" The suggested format helps decrease patient defensiveness when reporting psychosocial difficulties.

After inquiring about stresses, the physician can investigate sources of social support. For example:

Physician: Whom can you turn to for support?

REFERENCES

1. Billings JA, Stoeckle JD: *The clinical encounter: a guide to the medical interview and case presentation*, St Louis, ed 2, 1998, Mosby.
2. Cohen-Cole SA et al: Psychiatric education for internists: a randomized controlled comparison of two teaching models, *Psychosom Med* 44:122, 1982.
3. Clark WD, McIntyre JR: The generalist and alcoholism: dilemmas and progress. In Noble J, editor: *Textbook of general medicine and primary care*, ed 3, St Louis, Mosby, in Press.

4. Ewing JA: Detecting alcoholism: the CAGE questionnaire, *JAMA* 252:1905, 1984.
5. Clark W: Effective interviewing and intervention for alcohol problems. In Lipkin M Jr, Putnam SM, Lazare A, editors: *The medical interview: clinical care, education, and research,* New York, 1995, Springer.
6. Cole S, Levinson R, Saravay S: The biopsychosocial model of illness. In Stoudemire A, editor: *An introduction to human behavior,* ed 3, Philadelphia, 1998, JB Lippincott.

CHAPTER 13 Review of Systems

The review of systems is an important part of the medical history that allows the physician to survey the various bodily systems and uncover significant symptoms that may not have already been revealed in the history of the present illness or the elaboration of the medical history.

Because the review of systems is designed to screen an enormous array of possible problems, interviewing skill is required to gather data systematically and efficiently without missing important details. Most patients understand the point of this part of the interview and cooperate with the physician in completing it rapidly and efficiently. Because most information relevant to the patient's current problems will already have been elicited in the discussion of the present illness and the medical history, the review of systems should be possible to complete in 5 to 10 minutes for most patients. Some patients who demonstrate a "positive review of systems," however, find some way to report symptoms in virtually every organ system. Such patients have also been said to present a "laundry list of complaints" and can be frustrating to interview. In general, these patients need to be directed toward the goal of reporting common, recurrent, or troubling symptoms and omitting infrequent or mild symptoms.

Experienced physicians often complete the review of systems while performing the physical examination. Screening questions can be asked of the patient while the physician is examining the relevant body part. Although this method is efficient, the physician must ensure that the patient knows the physician is asking general screening questions. Some patients become anxious because they imagine that questions are being asked about some physical abnormality that has appeared on the physical examination.

Because of the complexity of the review of systems, however, beginning students generally need to complete this part of the interview before they examine the patient. To remember important topics, most students also find it helpful to consult a list of relevant questions while they are interviewing patients. Students may write key questions on a sheet of paper, on a clipboard, or on an index card to refer to while they interview patients. Students are soon able to develop their own systems for remembering relevant questions and will no longer need reminders.

In general, an efficient review of systems is organized around body systems. These are the organ systems that must be evaluated:

1. Skin
2. Eyes
3. Ears, nose, mouth, sinuses, and throat
4. Pulmonary
5. Cardiovascular
6. Digestive
7. Genitourinary
8. Hematologic
9. Immune
10. Endocrine
11. Musculoskeletal
12. Neurologic
13. Psychiatric

The patient should be told that a separate part of the evaluation process is about to begin and that the physician will screen a wide variety of organ systems and physical problems to see whether anything important was omitted in the interview so far.

> **Physician:** The next part of the interview is different. I'm going to ask you a series of standard questions about common medical problems that you may or may not have experienced. This is our way of making sure we don't miss something that might be important.

A few selected questions are listed as examples for each of the organ systems. As students gain experience, they will develop skill in evaluating the significance of symptoms uncovered in the review of systems and they will learn to recognize patterns of patient responses that require more detailed follow-up. Several general questions are asked for each organ system. Physicians can also give patients a short list of symptoms and ask them whether they have ever experienced any of the symptoms. Positive responses by patients then need to be followed by more focused questions inquiring about the details of the complaint. The following list of questions represents an acceptable approach for beginning students:

1. *Skin:* Do you have any problems with your skin? What about things like itching, rashes, or sores?
2. *Eyes:* Do you have any problems with your eyes? What about things like trouble seeing, itching eyes, halos around lights, or blurring?
3. *Ears, nose, mouth, sinuses, and throat:* Do you have trouble with your hearing or your ears? Do you have trouble with your mouth and throat, nose, or sinuses?

4. *Lungs:* Any problems with your lungs? What about things like shortness of breath, coughing, or chest pain?
5. *Cardiovascular:* Trouble with your heart? What about things like a racing heart, chest pain, or irregular beats?
6. *Digestive:* Do you have trouble with your stomach? What about things like stomach pain, trouble with your bowels, or nausea?
7. *Genitourinary:* Any trouble with your urine? What about things like painful or frequent urination, unusual color or smell? What problems have you had with your sexual organs and private parts?
8. *Hematologic:* Any trouble with easy bruising or bleeding?
9. *Immunologic:* Any trouble with infections?
10. *Endocrine:* Do you get colder or hotter than others around you do?
11. *Musculoskeletal:* How are your joints and muscles? What about things like pain, swelling, or weakness?
12. *Neurologic:* Any trouble with your sense of smell or taste? Any problems with weakness in your arms or legs or unusual feelings like "tingling"? Any trouble with balance or walking? Any trouble with memory?
13. *Psychiatric:* How have your nerves been? Any problems with anxiety or depression? Have you ever been the recipient of an unwanted physical or sexual assault?

It is important to highlight the special importance of the psychiatric review of systems. Many patients with unexplained physical complaints suffer from unrecognized depression or anxiety or are victims of current or previous physical or sexual abuse.[1-2] These patients typically use excessive health care resources before their underlying psychiatric disorders or abuse history is recognized and appropriately treated. Sadly, sometimes the psychiatric problems or abuse are never recognized. Thus, while many aspects of the review of systems described in this chapter are often omitted in actual practice, the three psychiatric screening questions should be included in every complete medical evaluation.

REFERENCES

1. Warshaw C, Alpert E: Integrating routine inquiry about domestic violence into daily practice (editorial), *Ann Intern Med* 131(8):619-620, 1999.
2. Kroenke K, Jackson JL, Chamberlin S: Depressive and anxiety disorders in patients presenting with physical complaints: clinical predictors and outcome, *Am J Med* 103(5):339-357, 1997.

CHAPTER

14 Mental Status

An evaluation of mental status belongs in every complete medical workup. As with the patient profile and social history, the recommendations in medical texts for the mental status examination are sometimes far different from what is actually incorporated into routine medical practice. Most medical texts present a complex discussion of the mental status evaluation.[1] However, few physicians routinely incorporate a "formal" mental status examination into their interviews, and most written evaluations of mental status in patients' charts refer to "orientation" only with statements like "oriented × 3" or "confused" or "disoriented."[2]

This chapter presents the rationale for including a brief mental status evaluation in every medical workup and presents a succinct version of the mental status evaluation that can be easily and efficiently adapted for routine office practice. Because many patients require more extensive cognitive testing, physicians can develop higher-order skills in this area by consulting other references.[3]

WHY EVERY MEDICAL WORKUP SHOULD INCLUDE A MENTAL STATUS EVALUATION

The mental status of every patient should be evaluated because physicians need to be aware of abnormalities in mental functioning. Poor memory or other cognitive problems can lead to unreliability in the data collection process. Furthermore, the mental status evaluation provides the data on which to base psychiatric diagnoses.

As pointed out in Chapter 2, mental illness is common in the general population (about 20% of the population over any 6-month period of time) and among patients seeking general medical care as well.[4]

Carefully conducted studies have revealed that 25% to 33% of primary care patients suffer from a mental disorder diagnosable by a structured psychiatric interview. Perhaps another 20% have significant emotional problems or symptoms complicating their physical illnesses.

Repeated research indicates that one third to one half of these psychiatric problems are not recognized by primary care physicians.[5]

Some students may wonder about the importance of recognizing mental disorders in their patients. They may believe that mentally ill patients really "belong" in the mental health sector of the health care system, and that it may not be appropriate for primary providers to explore such problems in their patients. However, there are several reasons that physicians should develop more skills in the recognition and management of mental disorders. First, 50% to 60% of the mentally ill patients in this country obtain their only mental health care from primary care providers.[6] Many mentally ill patients seek general medical attention because physical complaints are more "legitimate" avenues for the expression of psychiatric problems. Most psychiatric conditions are psychobiologic conditions in which physical complaints are common (e.g., sleep disorder in depression and palpitations or shortness of breath in panic disorder). Many patients focus on these physical symptoms when seeking medical attention rather than face the stigma of psychiatric care. Primary care patients with mental illness use twice as much nonpsychiatric medical care as patients without mental illness do.[7] Furthermore, most patients who eventually commit suicide seek some type of medical help in the weeks before their suicide.[8]

For general humanitarian reasons as well as public health and efficiency, physicians should increase their ability to recognize and manage psychiatric disorders that occur in their clinical and hospital practices. Developing proficiency in the use of a brief mental status examination is one important part of learning to recognize mental disorders.

In addition to affective and anxiety disorders that are often missed with medical patients, cognitive impairment is frequently overlooked, especially in hospitalized patients. One study in an inner-city hospital found that 33% of the medically ill patients had significant cognitive impairment and that with 50% of these patients the condition was unrecognized by their physicians.[9] It is important for physicians to recognize cognitive impairment because limited cognitive capacity can lead to inaccurate data collection by the physician and poor compliance. In addition, many cognitive problems are associated with treatable and sometimes reversible disorders.

BRIEF MENTAL STATUS EXAMINATION

Most parts of the brief mental status evaluation can be completed without asking the patient specific questions. Significant information about mental status is obtained throughout the interview process through careful observation of such things as the patient's general appearance and behavior, speech, thought process, judgment, recounting of medical history, and affect. The physician may need to ask the patient only three or four screening questions to complete the entire mental status examination as presented here. Thus the mental status examination is an ongoing process throughout the interview and may require only 3 or 4 minutes of special questioning by itself.

The brief mental status evaluation includes six basic categories. By convention, the oral presentation and written description of the mental status evaluation are included as the first part of the neurologic examination (part of the overall physical examination).

General Appearance and Behavior

The physician can make the general description of the patient without asking the patient any questions. The general description is a short statement about how the patient appears overall to the examiner. The general description should give the listener or reader a "snapshot" of the patient's presentation and should provide a great deal of information about the patient's general condition. Areas of concern are the patient's attention to or ability for self-care (neat? disheveled?) and rapport with the physician (cooperative? suspicious?). For the purposes of oral presentation or written documentation, the following description might be appropriate:

> ***Mr. Barnes was lying quietly in bed and appeared somewhat disheveled. He answered questions slowly and somewhat hesitantly.***

Speech

The quality and quantity of speech should be described. For example, speech can be rapid or slow, coherent or disorganized and rambling, or clear or slurred. The description of a patient's speech gives a great deal of information concerning emotional and neurologic functioning. The quality and quantity of speech can be observed without asking any specific questions:

> ***Mrs. Fander's speech was clear and coherent.***
> or
> ***Mr. Spikes's speech was slurred and rambling.***

Mood and Affect

"Mood" generally refers to an underlying emotional state, and "affect" describes more momentary modulation of feelings in the course of an interview. For the purposes of the brief mental status evaluation, it is not necessary to separate the two categories. In this section the physician should describe the predominant feeling tone communicated by the patient (e.g., sadness, anger, or anxiety). The patient occasionally demonstrates more than one significant feeling; when this occurs, the physician should record it. If the physician observes an inappropriate or flat affect, this should also be described. For example:

> ***Mr. Kline demonstrated appropriate affect throughout the interview but seemed quite anxious in discussing his test results.***
> or
> ***Mr. Blane seemed very depressed throughout the interview and cried several times as he discussed his difficulty in working.***

One or two screening questions can be productive for the evaluation of mood and affect. For example:

> **Physician:** How have you reacted to all these problems? How much stress or tension have you been feeling lately? How often do you feel sad or "blue"?

Thought Content

The evaluation of thought content refers to the patient's main concerns, the presence of psychotic phenomena like delusions, and the presence of suicidal or homicidal ideation. For the purposes of most medical interviews, the patient's main concern is the chief complaint and present illness, and there is no further need to ask questions. However, patients demonstrating emotional distress should be asked about suicidal ideation. Physicians should be reassured that this type of inquiry can be lifesaving and does not "put ideas" into patients' heads. Of course, concern and sensitivity to the patient's emotional concerns must be shown, and then the physician can sensitively ask a question such as the following:

> **Physician:** With all these problems you've been having, I wonder—do you ever think that life is not worth living?

With this type of introduction the physician can begin exploring the patient's specific thoughts and plans about possible suicide. These are higher-order skills and are addressed in detail in numerous other places.[10]

Cognition and Sensorium

This physician should describe patients' orientation and general mental functioning. The patient's sensorium refers to the ability to interact with the environment. Orientation to person, place, date, and situation (four separate dimensions) can be a rough proxy for sensorium. If a patient were fully oriented in all four spheres, it would be unusual for him or her to have an impairment in sensorium such that he or she could not interact meaningfully with the environment. Evaluating the cognitive status of every patient is essential. To minimize patient discomfort, this can be introduced as another part of the routine evaluation. For example:

> **Physician:** Mrs. Smith, I need to ask you a few questions about your memory and thinking. These are routine. Some are quite easy, and some may be more difficult. Where are you right now? What is today's date?

After the physician has asked the orientation questions, he or she should complete at least a brief cognitive screening. A short-term memory task and at least one other complex cognitive task is adequate for screening purposes. Patients can be asked to remember three objects after 3 minutes and to complete one more cognitive challenge that may be appropriate to their educational level. The physician can complete this test of short-term memory by asking the patient to repeat three specific words after the examiner has said them and then to remember them for a few minutes. For example:

> **Physician:** Now, Mr. Brown, I'm going to say three words, and I would like you to say them after me. Then I would like you to try to remember them in a few minutes. I will ask you for them again. The words are "house," "car," and "tree."

After the patient has registered the words, one complex cognitive task appropriate to educational level should be administered. For example, college-educated patients can be asked to subtract 7 from 100 and keep going for about 1 minute. If the patient is less well educated, suitable alternatives could be to spell "world" backward, subtract serial 3's from 100, recite the months of the year or days of the week backward, or recite seven numbers forward or four numbers backward, for example. Alternately, patients can be asked to draw the face of a clock, put in the numbers, and place the long and short arms of the clock at the appropriate place to indicate a specific time (e.g., 10 minutes before 2). After this task is complete, the patient can be asked to recall the three words.

In general, the brief mental status evaluation will take no more than 3 or 4 minutes for patients who do not have a significant mental disorder or significant cognitive impairment.

REFERENCES

1. Martin DC: The mental status examination. In Walker HK et al, editors: *The history, physical, and laboratory examinations,* Boston, 1990, Butterworths.
2. Cohen-Cole SA et al: Psychiatric education for internists: a randomized controlled comparison of two teaching models, *Psychosom Med* 44:122, 1982.

3. Manschrenck TC, Keller MB: The mental status examination. In Lazare A, editor: *Outpatient psychiatry: diagnosis and treatment*, Baltimore, 1989, Williams & Wilkins.
4. Shapiro S et al: Utilization of health and mental health services: three epidemiologic catchment area sites, *Arch Gen Psychiatry* 41:971-978, 1984.
5. Cole S, Saravay S, Levinson R: The biopsychosocial model of illness. In Stoudemire A, editor: *An introduction to human behavior*, ed 3, Philadelphia, 1997, JB Lippincott.
6. Regier DA, Narrow WE, Rae DS et al: The de facto U.S. mental and addictive disorders service system. Epidemiologic catchment area prospective 1-year prevalence rates of disorders and services, *Arch Gen Psych* 50:85-94, 1993.
7. Unetzer J, Patrick DL, Simon L, et al: Depressive symptoms and the cost of health services in HMO patients aged 65 years and older. A 4-year prospective study, *JAMA* 277(28):618-623, 1997.
8. Barraclough B, Bunelz J, Nelson B, et al: A hundred cases of suicide: clinical aspects, *Br J Psychiatry* 125:355-373, 1974.
9. Gehi et al: Is there a need for admission and discharge cognitive screening for the medically ill? *Gen Hosp Psychiatry* 3:186-191, 1980.
10. Cohen-Cole S, Mance R: Interviewing the suicidal patient. In Lipkin M Jr, Putnam S, Lazare A, editors: *The medical interview: clinical care, education, and research,* New York, 1995, Springer-Verlag.

UNIT IV

UNDERSTANDING THE PATIENT'S EMOTIONAL RESPONSES

CHAPTER

15 Normal Reactions

With few exceptions, illness generates emotional distress. In particular, chronic illness leads to a wide variety of negative emotional reactions as patients endure the many stresses of illness and struggle to meet the adaptive challenges posed by their illness. This chapter reviews the common stresses and related adaptive tasks. Physicians who understand these stresses and challenges will be better able to help patients cope with the emotions that often result.

COMMON STRESSES OF ILLNESS

Strain and Grossman[1] have described eight different stresses of illness. The list that follows represents a modification of their contributions.

Threat to Efficacy

Patients who are sick usually become less effective in the world. Self-esteem and a sense of value in the world derive in part from what a person is able to do. Illness interferes with this ability to perform effectively at a job, at home, or in leisure activities. If patients had been working, they often must cope with the loss of a job or the threat of the loss of a job. For patients who are homemakers, illness may compromise the ability to work in the home. Sickness may make it impossible for fathers to "roughhouse" with their children or take them fishing. Mothers may be unable to function in the ways that bring them pleasure or recognition from those around them.

Threat of Separation

Especially when the possibility of hospitalization is involved, illness can generate the fear of separation from people who are loved and who are perceived as needed for comfort and support. The enforced dependency of illness or hospitalization can reawaken early childhood separation fears.

Threat of Loss of Love

Many patients fear that illness will make them unattractive or unlovable to the people around them.

Threat of Loss of Body Function

Illness often leads to urinary or fecal incontinence. This is usually embarrassing to patients and sometimes terrifying. It makes a person feel like a baby, with all the associated and complex meanings that being babylike signifies to different individuals.

Threat of Loss of Body Parts

Sometimes patients are afraid (many times with good reason) that they might lose an important part of their body.

Threat of Loss of Rationality

Illness often compromises mental and cognitive functioning. Patients who are ill or who take medications may become more forgetful, may have trouble concentrating, or, in general, may lose some of their previous levels of mental control. The idea of "going crazy" terrifies many patients who do not realize that this cognitive loss is commonly associated with many physical illnesses and treatments.

Physicians can be quite helpful to patients by educating them with a simple statement such as the following:

> **Physician:** Many patients feel that they are losing their minds during some illnesses. This is a common problem, and the mental confusion you may be experiencing can be expected to clear in a few days.

Threat of Pain

In general, patients are afraid of pain and do not want to suffer.

ADAPTIVE TASKS OF ILLNESS

The stresses of illness described previously confront the patient with a host of challenges to which he or she must adapt. The consequences of good or poor adaptation have significant implications for the quality of life of the patient and for the type of care the physician attempts to administer.

Maintaining Emotional Balance

The stresses of illness lead to a variety of patients' emotional reactions that are described later in the chapter in more detail. Patients are faced with the challenge of experiencing these emotional dislocations and trying to weather them and continue with their lives. This is difficult and sometimes impossible to accomplish.

Preserving Social Relationships

Because illness creates so many complicated difficulties in many patients' lives, normal social relationships often become strained. The ability to sustain relationships in spite of illness is a core task for patients, especially those with chronic illness.

Preserving Family Relationships

Preserving family relationships can be even more difficult and important than maintaining social relationships in general. Sickness often alters relationships in the family; the breadwinner role may switch from the male to the female, and the homemaker role may switch from the female to the male. Patterns of intimacy, role responsibility, sexuality, and parenting can all be altered by chronic illness. A favorable outcome is usually associated with patients who are able to preserve their core relationships despite necessary alterations in social role functioning.

Coping with Disability

Illness is often associated with physical impairments that render some type of disability. Among the possible impairments are difficulty ambulating, physical pain, trouble using one's hands, difficulty seeing or hearing, trouble sleeping, inability to carry out activities of daily living, and inability to drive. Adapting to the physical impairments causing the disability is a continuing and sometimes overwhelming task for patients.

Coping with the Unknown

Many illnesses have an unpredictable course. Some patients may get better, some worse, and some stay about the same. Patients have to cope with this enormous uncertainty when predicting the future level of their physical impairment. Some patients do not know whether they will die from their current illness.

Coping with Pain

Pain is part of many illnesses; unfortunately, severe pain is common. Some patients must learn to live with this pain in a way that enables them to continue functioning in as productive a manner as possible.

Adapting to a Variety of Health Care Providers

Chronic illness requires patients to come into contact with a great variety of health care professionals. Patients must try to deal with many different physicians representing different specialties and with different individual temperaments as well. For example, nurses, secretaries, nutritionists, and physical therapists represent specialties and personalities to which the patient must try to adapt. This can be a manageable task for some and an impossible one for others.

"NORMAL" EMOTIONAL REACTIONS TO ILLNESS

As described previously, most patients experience a variety of emotional reactions to illness. While these vary from individual to individual and from disease to disease, there are some predictable and common emotional stages that the physician should understand and recognize. Once they are understood, the physician may be able to respond more effectively and helpfully to patients.

Regression

Regression refers to the psychic phenomenon of reliance on more childlike stages of emotional functioning in response to illness. This universal response to illness encourages increased physical and emotional dependency during illness. For the most part, limited regression can be adaptive, to permit rest and recovery from acute illnesses or during exacerbations of chronic illness. Indeed, our health care system values this dependency to some extent because being a "good" patient is often perceived as doing what the doctor says without question.

Chronic illness demands severe limitations on this regression and dependency. Functioning in the face of chronic illness often requires considerable effort on both the physician's and patient's parts to overcome the regressive tendencies of illness. Patients respond differently to this dependency; some patients find it hard to relinquish, and others find any dependency at all to be extremely threatening.

Denial, Suppression, and Repression

One of the initial emotional reactions to news about an illness is the absence of an observable emotion. The consequences and emotional impact of an illness may be so great that many patients deny the news.

Denial can take many forms. When the patient simply pushes the idea of the illness out of his or her mind and manages to avoid thinking about it, this coping mechanism can actually contribute to better functioning. Technically, this is called *suppression,* which is considered a relatively healthy type of defense mechanism. The thoughts are still on the borders of consciousness, but the patient is able to divert his or her attention from the problem for short periods.

Repression refers to the unintentional movement of a thought from consciousness to unconsciousness. This can be adaptive in some circumstances, but it can also lead to negative consequences, such as forgetting to keep appointments and forgetting medicine.

Denial is potentially the most deleterious of this group of defenses, in which the information received from physicians is contradicted. If a patient is told he or she has cancer, the patient who denies this information insists that the physician is wrong.

Typical problems related to denial appear in patients with coronary artery disease who insist that their chest pain symptoms are "heartburn" and not heart disease, because they cannot face the implications of having a heart attack. Unfortunately, this type of denial can be life threatening when it leads to a delay in the time it takes for patients to receive treatment.

Anxiety

Anxiety is, of course, another common and expected part of almost all illnesses, and almost every ill patient experiences at least some degree of anxiety. For the purposes of this text, anxiety and fear are not distinguished. Anxiety refers to the subjective experience of fear, dread, and foreboding. This can take many forms and vary in intensity throughout the course of any illness. Each of the stresses and threats described previously is usually associated with some fearful reactions on the part of the patient.

Patients can experience anxiety as an internal state of fearfulness, but the anxiety can also have somatic manifestations and influence the course of the primary physical illness. For example, anxiety can cause autonomic nervous system activation such as palpitations, gastrointestinal hypermotility, sweating, and sleeplessness. When anxiety is unrelieved, it can exert a negative influence on the disease process. At times, anxiety becomes so intense and pervasive that it actually becomes an independent psychiatric condition. (This situation is reviewed in Chapter 16.)

Anger

Anger, too, is a common concomitant of chronic illness. Patients wonder, "Why me?" They are often angry with their God or feel spiritual uncertainty as they try to understand the ultimate meaning of the illness. This commonly leads to anxiety, as well as to anger.

Many patients feel a generalized anger that cannot be focused on any one particular idea or person. When this occurs, they often lash out unexpectedly and seemingly without good reason at everyone around them. Physicians and other medical providers are typical targets, as are valued friends and family. This is unfortunate, since some angry patients alienate the people they most need for support during physical and emotional crises. However, when made aware of these reactions, medical providers and family can often deal with them better with fewer maladaptive consequences for the patient.

Sadness

Sadness is a common reaction to any illness. In fact, physicians would suspect the "normalcy" of anyone who becomes chronically ill and does not experience sadness. Chronic illness usually leads to many losses—such as loss of work function, leisure pleasures, physical pleasures, and relationships. Sadness is the most common and expected emotional reaction to loss, although other reactions such as anger and anxiety also play a role in loss.

However, sadness is not the same as persistent, clinically significant major depression. This distinction will be highlighted in more detail in Chapter 16. In brief, a normal sad reaction to illness will not color every aspect of a person's relationship with those around him or her. "Normal" sadness still allows the anticipation and experience of pleasurable activities over time, even if they are extremely limited when compared with previous activities. Clinical depression, on the other hand, pervades every aspect of life, to the extent that the patient can no longer experience any interest or pleasure in living.

REFERENCES

1. Strain JJ, Grossman S: Psychological reactions to medical illness and hospitalization. In Strain JJ, Grossman S, editors: *Psychological care of the medically ill: a primer in liaison psychiatry*, 1975, New York, Appleton.

CHAPTER

16 Maladaptive Reactions

The various emotional responses to illness that were discussed in Chapter 15 could be considered "normal" in the sense that most individuals facing chronic or serious illness experience them to some degree. However, even more important than the statistical normality of these emotions is that they can be considered normal when they themselves do not disrupt a patient's overall quality of life. On the other hand, for many patients these emotional responses begin to interfere with functioning. In such cases these reactions can rightly be considered "maladaptive."

In general, the concept of maladaptive responses to illness is more useful to patients and physicians than is the concept of "abnormality." The idea of an abnormal emotional reaction conveys such a pejorative tone that physicians and patients shrink from accepting such a label. This text therefore urges the use of functional terms such as "adaptive" and "maladaptive" to describe emotional reactions to illness.

Emotions can be considered maladaptive when they interfere with a patient's quality of life or overall functioning. There are many types of maladaptive emotional responses, and sometimes these take the form of mixed emotional reactions. This chapter focuses on three basic types of response sets that can develop into relatively fixed patterns of maladaptive behavior: anger, depression, and anxiety.

PERSISTENT ANGER

As was discussed in the previous chapter, most patients with a chronic illness become angry at some point in the coping process. Patients often ask bitterly, "Why me? What did I do to deserve this sickness?" The anger can take the form of lashing out at family members, at physicians, or at anyone who happens to be around. It is often helpful for physicians to remember that this inappropriate anger, at times directed at them, may be a displacement of the anger that the patient feels about the illness itself.

Anger can become seriously maladaptive when it is so persistent and offensive that the patient alienates the people he or she most needs for physical and emotional support. The patient can be so unpleasant that nurses and physicians stay away. This can lead to more angry demands for attention and to further isolation. Thus the angry response may lead to a self-defeating circle of angry demands and withdrawal of staff. In addition, the anger may cover up underlying fear.

The angry patient may alienate friends and family. For example, when receiving visitors, an angry patient may demand to know why they came and may insinuate ulterior motives rather than graciously accepting whatever sympathy and concern the visitors offer. Such attitudes can lead to even more isolation and loneliness than the physical illness itself might cause. In addition, this apparent social rejection can contribute to an already low sense of self-esteem.

ADJUSTMENT DISORDER WITH DEPRESSED MOOD AND MAJOR DEPRESSION

Most serious or chronic illnesses lead to sadness. This is certainly an expected response. However, some patients develop persistent despondent feelings that interfere with their ability to work, to function in social roles, or to relate to the important people in their lives. When sadness becomes this severe, current psychiatric nomenclature would probably describe such patients as meeting diagnostic criteria either for an adjustment disorder with depressed mood or for a major depression.[1]

An adjustment disorder with depressed mood is defined as an emotional response (i.e., a sad response) to a stressful life event that is stronger and more persistent than would be expected in most individuals. Major depression, on the other hand, describes a syndromal set of signs and symptoms including at least 2 weeks of persistent unhappiness or anhedonia (pervasive loss of interest or pleasure). A characteristic set of physical signs (poor sleep, loss of appetite, fatigue, and psychomotor agitation or retardation) and psychologic symptoms (poor concentration, low self-esteem or guilt, and hopelessness) constitutes the syndrome of major depression. In general, major depression is best conceptualized as a psychobiologic illness. It tends to occur in genetically predisposed individuals and may develop in response to significant life stressors.[2] Depending on the individual and the biologic substrate, these stressors may need to be extraordinarily potent or in some cases may be rather minor. In fact, with sufficient biologic loading, major depression may appear in the absence of any discernible stressor.[3]

Some physicians and patients tend to explain away a major depression by saying things like, "Anyone with this condition would be depressed." While this statement might be true in the sense that anyone with the condition would be sad, it is not true that everyone with a serious illness develops major depression. Studies of terminally ill cancer patients, as well as studies of patients with other serious illnesses, indicate that fewer than half of such patients demonstrate the signs and symptoms of major depression.

Patients who develop major depression in the context of a significant and chronic physical illness develop levels of functional impairment that far exceed the impairment expected from the physical illness itself. Relationships are damaged, the ability to function is impaired, and the overall quality of life is grossly decreased. This maladaptive response to illness is important to recognize because in many instances it can be effectively treated. Therefore, major depression occurring in the context of a physical illness should always be considered a "dread complication" of the illness that needs immediate and aggressive treatment rather than an expected reaction that cannot be treated.

ADJUSTMENT DISORDER WITH ANXIOUS MOOD/ANXIETY DISORDERS

Anxiety is the third general type of maladaptive response to illness. As pointed out in Chapter 15, some degree of anxiety is a typical response to most illnesses. Patients are usually anxious about the meaning of the illness in their lives and about how the illness will affect their life as the illness progresses. Anxiety is thus common and expected.

Persistent anxiety is disabling by itself and interferes with the coping process, as well as with physical recovery. Patients with persistent anxiety cannot separate themselves from their fears. They cling to doctors, friends, and family with persistent questions that often cannot be answered and demands that cannot be met. They may suffer from autonomic system activation with tachycardia, sweating, diarrhea, cramps, shortness of breath, hyperventilation, and trouble sleeping. When patients suffer from persistent anxiety in the face of chronic illness, physicians must recognize the condition and treat it properly. Persistent anxiety may meet criteria for adjustment disorder with anxious mood, panic disorder, or generalized anxiety disorder.[1]

An adjustment disorder with anxious mood is nosologically similar to an adjustment disorder with depressed mood. The name of this condition refers to a case in which an individual reacts to a stressor with an emotional reaction that exceeds what might be expected in most individuals. In this case the reaction is marked more by tension, fear, and nervousness than by depression. On the other hand, panic disorder is a severe psychiatric condition marked by unpredictable attacks of sudden panic that are often characterized by a sense of impending doom, hyperventilation, chest pain, sweating, and so on. Panic attacks are often associated with agoraphobia (a fear of going outside).

A generalized anxiety disorder, on the other hand, is a severe anxiety disorder marked by 6 months of significant anxiety symptoms, including autonomic arousal (e.g., hyperventilation and palpitations) and fearful behavior toward the environment (e.g., vigilance and scanning).

INTERVIEWING STRATEGIES FOR PATIENTS WITH MALADAPTIVE EMOTIONAL RESPONSES

In general, interviews with patients who demonstrate maladaptive emotional responses require skills that are of a higher order than the ones described so far in this text. Despite this need for higher-order skills, the interventions presented in Chapter 3 are often helpful for patients who are angry, depressed, or anxious. However, when these emotional responses have become solidified into persistent patterns, the basic skills can only serve as a useful starting point for interaction, and further efforts and skills are usually necessary. A few principles are presented below, but the interested reader can consult other references for more detailed discussion of these topics.[4]

Persistently Angry Patients

Some angry patients respond to reflection and legitimation, as discussed in Chapter 3. Consider the following case:

> ***Mr. Bailes is a 56-year-old construction worker in the intensive care unit with arrhythmias after an acute myocardial infarction. He is enraged because the nurses will not allow him to get out of bed to use the bedside commode. His anger seems to be leading to excitement, which itself can exacerbate the arrhythmias.***

The physician might say the following:

Physician: Mr. Bailes, I can see that you are pretty upset. (reflection)

Patient: I sure am. Wouldn't you be upset if they wouldn't let you out of bed to take a crap? I don't mind pissing into a jug, but this bedpan thing won't do. There's a toilet five feet from my bed, and they won't let me out.

Physician: I'm not sure exactly how I would feel, but I can understand that this is really making you miserable. (legitimation) Can you tell me a little more about the ways in which it bothers you?

By reflecting and legitimating the patient's feelings, the physician can build a therapeutic alliance and let the patient ventilate his or her frustration. After this has occurred, the physician can compromise and negotiate to help the angry patient cooperate more fully with a treatment plan. Often the compromises must include concessions by the health care team to achieve any level of patient cooperation. The intensive care unit patient discussed above felt so humiliated by enforced dependency on a bedpan that the staff decided to let him use the bedside commode, even though this was not the most desirable solution from a narrow biologic point of view.

Some patients remain angry even after the physician has attempted to listen and let them ventilate their feelings by using skills such as reflection, legitimation, or any others available to the physician. Higher-order skills, consultations with supervisors or colleagues, and psychiatric consultation should all be considered at that time.

Patients Who Have an Adjustment Disorder With Depressed Mood or Major Depression

The sad or depressed patient can also be approached by using reflection and legitimation at first.

> *Mr. Gaines is a 62-year-old businessman who has chronic pulmonary disease and feels despondent about returning to work. When asked about the effect of the illness on his life, he weeps.*

The physician can say something such as this:

> **Physician:** I see this is quite overwhelming to you. (reflection)
>
> **Patient:** I'm just so upset, I don't know what to do. I can't sleep and I don't have any appetite. Nothing seems important anymore. I think I'm going to have to give up my business. (He begins to cry.)
>
> **Physician:** I can understand why that would be very upsetting. We're going to do everything we can to help you get better and also to help you with these bad feelings you've been having. (legitimation and support)

While empathy from the physician often helps such a patient momentarily, this patient's depression may be so severe that psychotherapy, antidepressant medication, or psychiatric consultation may be necessary.

Patients Who Have an Adjustment Disorder With Anxious Mood or an Anxiety Disorder

Anxiety as an example of a maladaptive emotional response is considered in the following patient:

> *Ms. James is a 21-year-old married female with a congenital liver problem and need for a transplant. She has always been anxious,*

but now her anxiety is disabling, and she is so afraid of surgery that she may not be able to undergo the operation.

The physician may pursue the interview in the following way:

Physician: I'd like to know more about how you've been feeling lately.
Patient: Doctor, I'm scared about the surgery. My palms are sweaty all the time, I can't sleep, and I've got butterflies in my stomach.
Physician: I see you're anxious. (reflection) Maybe you can tell me some more about your specific worries.
Patient: I'm worried about what the operation will be like. I don't know who will take care of my kids. I'm afraid I won't do well after the surgery. And I've been getting more of these panic spells I've been treated for before.
Physician: You have a lot of reasons to be anxious. (legitimation) I'm going to do what I can to help you figure out what you can expect from your surgery, and I also want to help you deal with some of your anxious feelings. (support)

While the appropriate use of reflection, legitimation, and support, as well as other skills, can all help the anxious patient, some patients may still need more extensive interventions. Patients suffering from significant anxiety symptoms or an anxiety disorder generally require a physician with higher-order skills to diagnose problems accurately and to provide appropriate therapeutic support or appropriate antianxiety medication. Psychiatric referral may also be indicated.

REFERENCES

1. American Psychiatric Association: *Diagnostic and statistical manual of mental disorders, IV*, Washington, D.C., 1994, American Psychiatric Association Press.
2. Cole S, Raju M, Barret J, et al: The MacArthur Foundation Depression Education Program for Primary Care Physicians: background, participants' workbook, and facilitator's guide, *General Hospital Psychiatry*, in press.
3. Rush AS, Golden WE, Moll EC, et al: *Depression in primary care: clinical practice guidelines*, Agency for Healthcare Policy and Research Publication no. 93-0550, Rockville, Md, 1993, U.S. Department of Health and Human Services.
4. Novack DH: Therapeutic aspects of the clinical encounter (review), *J Gen Intern Med* 2(5):346-355, 1987.

UNIT

V

MANAGING COMMUNICATION CHALLENGES

CHAPTER

17 Sexual Issues in the Interview

Sexual issues in the interview merit a separate chapter because these concerns are such an important but generally neglected dimension of general medical care. Medical students and practicing physicians tend to avoid discussion of sexual issues for understandable reasons. Sex is a "private matter" and the locus of powerful emotions that can cause great distress, shame, and humiliation. Students and physicians tend to follow the natural tendency to avoid subjects that bear the risk of great embarrassment to themselves or their patients. Because of the importance of sexuality to health and illness, however, avoiding these issues leads to bad medical care. Developing good interviewing skills regarding sexuality requires intellectual and emotional effort.

Why Are Sexual Issues Important?

In the world of the human immunodeficiency virus (HIV) and acquired immunodeficiency syndrome (AIDS), it is no longer difficult to convince medical students that interviewing about sexuality is important to medical care. Because of the prevalence and severity of these conditions, it is now clear that every patient must be evaluated and educated about HIV and AIDS. However, even without the importance of this epidemic, interviewing about sexuality remains a core dimension of the doctor-patient relationship.

Besides HIV and AIDS, numerous other sexually transmitted diseases (STDs) cause significant morbidity and mortality. Physicians must understand these conditions and develop the ability to obtain appropriate information in the interview to assess risk.

The importance of interviewing about sexuality goes far beyond the ability to assess and manage STDs. Most important, sexuality is one of the core dimensions of a patient's quality of life. Primary sexual disorders are common (e.g., anorgasmia and impotence), and sexual dysfunction secondary to chronic physical illnesses or its treatment (e.g., spinal cord injury, coronary artery disease, hypertension, and depression) is almost universal.

Few patients with chronic illness escape the sexual problems commonly associated with the condition or its treatment. Typical problems include decreased libido or decreased competence (e.g., impaired erection, impaired ejaculation, or impaired orgasmic function). These issues can result from illness or the medication used to treat the illness. Patients do not typically discuss these problems unless physicians ask about them. Unfortunately, these sexual dysfunctions often lead to a significant impairment in the quality of life and to relationship problems with a spouse or a significant other.

Sexual problems often become crucial to determining patients' overall adjustment to their illnesses. Evaluation of sexual dysfunction thus becomes one of the core competencies of good medical interviewing.

In general, interviewing regarding sexual issues is most effective when the basic skills of the three-function model are applied to the sexual dimension of health and illness.

FUNCTION ONE: BUILDING THE RELATIONSHIP

Because interviewing about sexuality has the potential to cause great embarrassment, it is usually helpful for the student or physician to address potential emotional discomfort even before difficult subjects are raised. For example, in introducing discussion about sexuality, the physician might say something such as the following:

Physician: I need to ask you some questions now about your sexual life. These questions often make patients uncomfortable, but I need to assure you that these questions are a routine part of the medical evaluation. I ask them of all my patients, and they often provide information that is important to good medical care.

With this type of introduction, most patients will be able to discuss their sexual life without great distress. If it becomes clear that the patient is uncomfortable, the physician can use the relationship skills discussed earlier in the text: reflection, legitimation, support, partnership, and respect. For example:

Physician: I see these questions are making you uncomfortable. (reflection)
This is understandable. (legitimation)
Most people do find them difficult. (legitimation)
I appreciate your efforts to be open. (respect)
You should understand that I am only asking about what I consider to be important for your medical care. (support)
Do you think you and I can proceed along this line a bit further to

complete what is needed for a thorough medical assessment? (partnership)

Building the relationship is important for successful interviewing about sexual issues. If the patient does not feel comfortable or agree to this line of questioning, it is generally useless for the student or physician to proceed; without a cooperative patient, the information obtained will be suspect—either incomplete or incorrect. Thus relationship building must continue until the physician has a willing partner.

FUNCTION TWO: ASSESSING THE PROBLEM

Efficient and effective data gathering about sexuality requires the use of the same skills discussed earlier in the text: open-ended questioning, facilitation, surveying, and checking. Because of the sensitive nature of these topics, the skilled interviewer usually relies more heavily on attentive silence (as a facilitative technique), surveying, and specific closed-ended questions. The content of data gathering about sexual issues generally falls into one of two domains: (1) basic evaluation of risk (for STDs, primary sexual problems, use of protection, and history of abuse); and (2) evaluation of the impact of chronic illness on the sexual quality of life.

Basic Evaluation of Risk

A basic evaluation of risk (for STDs, primary sexual problems, use of protection, and history of sexual abuse) is now considered a standard part of the routine medical examination. Because these topics raise such anxiety for medical students and sometimes for patients, a separate chapter has been added to discuss the challenging dimensions of this interview process.

As discussed previously, the physician should lessen anxiety before beginning this line of questioning by making it clear that he or she asks all patients these questions. Questions about sexuality should begin in an open-ended manner and proceed to closed-ended questioning for purposes of clarification. Attentive silence is a particularly useful facilitative technique to help patients overcome their reluctance to speak about potentially embarrassing issues. Surveying about potential sexual issues is also a useful technique. Finally, specific closed-ended questions may become necessary to determine the specific information that is needed.

Throughout the sexual interview the physician should monitor the patient's emotional responses closely. Whenever questions seem to increase the patient's anxiety, the interview should address this anxiety directly. In general, complete medical interviews should include an evaluation of the patient's sexual orientation, sexual history, exposure to STDs, and use of protection during sexual intercourse, as well as a screening for sexual problems. Because of emerging data linking childhood sexual abuse with later unexplained physical complaints, patients should also be screened for a history of sexual abuse.

Physician: As I mentioned earlier, I need to ask you some questions about your sexual life that sometimes cause patients some embarrassment. I need to assure you that these are questions I ask everyone and that the information I may obtain may be important for your medical care. (Function one)
Can we start with your telling me something about your sexual life? (Function two)

In response to an open-ended question like this, patients frequently answer with a question, asking the physician to be more specific. For example:

Patient: What is it that you would like to know?
Physician: (Depending on the age, sex, or interview situation, the physician can use one or more of the following suggestions. If the patient has a chronic illness or specific symptoms, a useful opening often focuses on discussing the impact of the illness or symptoms on the patient's sexual life.)
Can you tell me how this illness has affected your sexual life?
or
Can you tell me a bit about your sexual life . . . tell me about your partner or partners?

Surveying can be helpful in the domain of sexual interviewing:

Physician: Perhaps you can tell me if you have any issues, concerns, or problems regarding your sexual life.

Attentive and supportive silence is particularly valuable after a question like this because the patient typically needs a few moments to make a decision to disclose potentially embarrassing information. In response to a combination of open-ended questioning, surveying, and attentive silence, most patients give the physician some basic information that can guide the physician's follow-up questions.

Eventually open questioning will need to be followed by closed questioning to obtain very specific answers to very specific and sometimes embarrassing questions. For example:

Physician: This information you have given me is very helpful. I do need to ask some more specific questions now.

How often have you had unprotected sexual intercourse in the last two years?
How many different sexual partners have had you in the last two years?
Have you experienced any difficulties in your sexual desire or activity in the last two years?
Have you ever experienced any unwelcome sexual advances, perhaps long ago in your childhood?

Impact of Chronic Illness on Sexual Quality of Life

Since most patients with chronic illness experience sexual dysfunction and are embarrassed to discuss it, it can be particularly helpful when initiating data gathering to detoxify the issue by "normalizing" dysfunction. For example:

Physician: As we discussed previously, discussion of sexual issues can cause some embarrassment, but it is an important part of the medical evaluation. Let me begin by pointing out that most patients with the type of illness you have experience some sexual difficulties. What difficulties have you been having?

Because sexual issues are sensitive, judicious use of facilitation becomes important. Attentive silence, head nodding, and the use of phrases such as "uh-huh" and "tell me more" are important skills to use at this point. Because patients give sensitive information only in small chunks, checking about information received is useful to make sure that information is accurate, but checking itself also serves as a facilitative technique for obtaining more information from the patient. For example:

Physician: Let me see if I understand you correctly. You said that you have noticed that the chest pain seems to have gotten in the way of your sexual life. You don't seem to have intercourse as often as you did before your illness began. Can you tell me more about . . .?

Clarification is essential in interviewing about sexuality because embarrassment often leads to vagueness. Physicians must become very concrete to help their patients be specific. For example:

Physician: I do understand your point about the decreasing frequency of intercourse. But it would help me understand you better if you could be more specific. How often were you and your partner having sexual intercourse before you got sick and how often are you having relations now?

Many patients with chronic illnesses notice that sexual issues, among other problems, can impair their relationships with their partners. This can lead to a crucial loss of social support, which in itself is a risk factor for further morbidity and mortality. It is important for physicians to assess these potential problem areas:

Physician: You have told me a little about the sexual problems that have emerged, as a result of this illness. How have these problems interfered with your general relationship with your wife?

FUNCTION THREE: MANAGING THE PROBLEMS

Efficient and effective education, negotiation, and adherence management for sexual issues and problems rely on the same basic interviewing skills discussed earlier in the text. Because of the delicacy of these concerns, however, special attention needs to be paid to patient understanding and patient commitment. Physicians need to regularly check the patient's understanding and commitment. Physicians should not say things such as, "Do you understand what I have been saying?" or, "Remember to practice safe sex, OK?" It is far better to use checking and to explicitly elicit a statement of commitment from the patient:

Physician To make sure that I have communicated clearly, could you please review for me what I have been telling you about safe-sex techniques?

or

To make sure that you and I have reached an understanding, please review for me what you are willing to commit yourself to doing, regarding safe-sex techniques.

Managing the Interviewer's Anxiety or Attitudinal Barriers

Interviewing about sexual issues causes all students and physicians significant anxiety. This anxiety is normal. Students and physicians are simply not accustomed to asking people intimate details about their sexual lives. The difficulty of sexual interviewing varies among individuals, depending on personal psychology. Most individuals find that sexual interviewing of older patients of the opposite sex is particularly difficult. For example, this may seem to some interviewers as if they are asking their parents about their sexual lives. Some interviewers find it difficult to conduct sexual interviews with a patient to whom they feel attracted. For example, some male interviewers may find it difficult to interview (or examine) attractive young women. Mastering this anxiety requires first of all an attitude of acceptance and understanding. This anxiety is common. The interviewer must take the attitude that this is a standard part of clinical practice and must learn to develop appropriate emotional distance and appropriate professionalism. Many students and physicians bring personal biases about sexual orientation or behavior to their work with patients. Such prejudice should not be part of medical care. In fairness to their patients, students or physicians who are burdened with negative attitudes should use self-examination and discussion with colleagues or teachers to overcome these barriers to unbiased care.

The only way to master the anxiety or other barriers associated with sexually oriented interviewing and to achieve a high level of skill is to practice. Role play is a convenient and effective way to practice interviewing about sexuality. Using role play to practice interviewing skills, with feedback from instructors and peers, offers an unequaled opportunity to gain proficiency and to master anxiety or other barriers.

Management of Specific Problems

Numerous sexual problems require intervention by the physician. A failure to practice safe sex (as discussed previously) is only one example. Others include the patient who is suffering from sexual problems related to illness (for example, the stroke patient with physical obstacles to intercourse), the patient with decreased arousal secondary to the use of antidepressant medication, or the patient who is currently at risk for sexual abuse. Physicians must develop a knowledge of initial management strategies (including knowledge of when, how, and where to make appropriate referrals) for these and other common sexual problems. A discussion of specific management approaches is beyond the scope of this text. However, the interviewing skills necessary to uncover the problems need to be acquired at an early stage of every medical career.

CONCLUSION

Interviewing about sexuality and sexual problems remains a complex and difficult dimension of the medical interview for students and physicians. Understanding the importance of this topic and relying on the basic skills of the three-function model can help most beginning interviewers become adept in this domain. In particular, use of initial rapport-building techniques to establish partnership, along with the use of attentive silence, surveying, direct questioning, and checking, can help interviewers reach a high level of competence in sexually oriented interviewing.

CHAPTER

18 Interviewing Elderly Patients

Interviewing elderly patients presents particular challenges to the beginning student, as it also does for physicians in practice. In particular, common patient disabilities and problems such as hearing or vision loss, cognitive impairment, social isolation, and physical impairment present obstacles that must be overcome to have a successful interview with the elderly patient.

Careful and sensitive application of the basic skills of the three-function model can meet most of the complex challenges associated with interviewing elderly patients. This chapter examines each of the three functions separately, with analysis of the ways the basic skills can be applied to maximize efficiency and effectiveness in the interview with elderly patients.

FUNCTION ONE: BUILDING RAPPORT WITH THE ELDERLY PATIENT

Since elderly patients often find the medical setting cumbersome, insensitive, and unresponsive to their needs, it is often helpful to anticipate this difficulty, to screen for elderly patients' frustrations early in the interview, and to take a few extra moments to build initial rapport. Even a few moments finding out patients' experiences with the health care system and listening to their difficulties can be particularly revealing and help cement the relationship for the future. An effort should be made to understand the patients' predicaments and empathize with their personal troubles. The skills of reflection, legitimation, support, partnership, and respect should be used. The worth of the initial investment of a few extra minutes in this endeavor will be the efficiency it will bring later.

A physician recently saw an elderly patient with Parkinson's disease and depression. The patient began the interview by noting that he had had numerous bad experiences with physicians and the health care system. The physician listened attentively and used rapport-building skills liberally in the initial 5 minutes. While this patient had numerous criticisms of other physicians whom he had seen previously, the interviewer did not have to join in this

criticism in order to build rapport. Straightforward empathic communication was usually sufficient:

Physician: It certainly seems like you have had some troubling experiences with the medical system. (reflection)
I can understand how you felt insignificant and unimportant. (legitimation)
I want you to know that I care about your difficulties and I will do the very best I can to work with you to develop a plan to bring you some relief. (support and partnership)

These relatively brief relationship-building interventions led to a meaningful, long-lasting relationship with this patient. The sense of caring communicated by this brief exchange facilitated the development of trust that was essential to ensure optimal clinical outcomes.

To build rapport with the elderly, the physician must meet with and build a relationship with the caregivers and family. When conflict or difficulty arises, it is important to meet with the significant others and listen to their difficulties too. Again, the initial investment in relationship building will pay enormous dividends later. For example:

Physician: (to caregiver) I would like to hear your thoughts on how your husband (father, grandfather . . .) is doing. And how has it been for you?
Family member: Well, it has been very difficult.
Physician: I can certainly understand why this has been so hard. I think you've been doing a terrific job coping with these problems, under the circumstances. (respect)

FUNCTION TWO: ASSESSING THE ELDERLY PATIENT

The assessment of the elderly patient uses the same skills that are used in assessing younger patients. When multiple disabilities and dysfunction come into play, however, more thoughtful attention to use of the basic skills becomes increasingly important. Careful listening is essential. With the elderly patient, as with all patients, the physician must use open-ended questions, facilitation, surveying, and checking. Because the prevalence of cognitive impairment increases with age, all elderly patients must receive the cognitive screen as part of the mental status examination (see Chapter 14). Pointing out that questions about orientation and memory are routine for all patients can help diffuse patient anxiety and resistance.

For many reasons, checking and summarizing are particularly important in interviews with the elderly. Because of hearing, vision, cognitive, or communication difficulties, elderly patients may not succeed in transmitting information accurately to the physician the first time. Similarly, when cognitive deficits may be present, checking information received helps confirm the reliability of the information. Checking is important with the elderly because the narratives of their medical histories are generally complex. These complexities multiply the possibilities for errors, misunderstandings, and omissions.

Given the potential problems of the interview, the interviewer of the elderly should take sufficient time to check his or her accurate understanding of the problem(s). This can save enormous time down the road. Checking is the most important data-gathering skill to use with the elderly. For example:

> **Physician:** With so much going on in your life, let me repeat back to you what I have just heard in order to make sure I have understood your problems correctly.

After relying on the skill of checking, the interviewer should pay special attention to the family and caregivers as sources of key information. An adequate assessment of the elderly patient must always include input from the family.

> **Physician:** (to family) I have spent some time with your spouse (father, grandmother . . .). Please let me know how you think she's been doing.

FUNCTION THREE: MANAGING THE PROBLEMS

Just as the first two functions require some particular attention and focus, so too does the third function when dealing with elderly patients. Patient education, negotiation, and adherence management require careful use of all the skills discussed earlier in this text. For elderly patients with significant disabilities, however, special attention to some of the basic skills becomes particularly pertinent. Perhaps the most important management skill for the elderly is *checking of understanding:*

> **Physician:** Just to make sure I have made myself clear, could you repeat back to me what I have told you about your condition?
> *or*
> Just to make sure we are together on the plan, could you repeat back to me what you are planning to do about your condition?

When it comes to management, the role of the family or caregiver is just as essential as it is for the successful completion of functions one and two, relationship building and assessment. Adherence increases whenever the family is involved in treatment planning.

Physician: I would like to make sure that everyone in the family understands what Mr. Gardner and I are planning for his condition . . .

CONCLUSION

Efficient and effective interviewing of elderly patients involves particular focus on and attention to some of the same skills that are recommended for use with younger patients: early development of rapport, checking of information and understanding, and involvement of the family throughout.

Because of elderly patients' high levels of anxiety and frustration with the medical system, early and systematic empathic interventions are essential to building effective rapport. The frequency of multiple disabilities necessitates checking to corroborate details of data gathering. To enhance understanding and adherence, physicians should rely again on checking to verify that the essential facts have been communicated and that patients are likely to follow the treatment plan.

In all stages of interviewing elderly patients, physicians must also involve the family or caregivers for maximum efficiency and effectiveness. Effective relationship building, accurate assessment, and pragmatic management depend on family and caregiver involvement from the beginning of the care process.

Successful interviewing of the elderly also requires patience and overcoming the students' or physicians' own attitudinal barriers. Students and physicians with biases against the elderly should use self-examination and discussion with peers and teachers to overcome these attitudinal barriers to unbiased care. Approaching the elderly with respect and focused attention to the skills emphasized in this chapter can minimize the time (and sometimes frustration) associated with interviewing the elderly and maximize physician, patient, and family satisfaction as well as clinical outcomes.

CHAPTER

19 Overcoming Cultural and Language Barriers

David J. Steele

This chapter provides general guidelines to help the physician maximize his or her effectiveness as a culturally sensitive medical interviewer. It also describes specific strategies for interacting with patients who are members of cultures different from those of the physician. Finally, this chapter addresses the challenges of using interpreters to interview patients who do not speak English. The premise underlying this chapter has been well stated by Johnson and his colleagues[1]:

> ***The overall goal of culturally sensitive care should be empathic understanding of the relationships among symptoms, distress, and the interpersonal life of the patient. One should show clear consideration of these culturally mediated personal meanings in the course and treatment of illness.***

Meeting the objectives of the three core interview functions—building rapport, assessing the patient, and managing the patient—requires the physician to be alert to the cultural beliefs and explanatory illness models influencing the patient's behavior. Once the physician has elicited and understood the patient's beliefs and behaviors, he or she is in a much better position to make effective use of the specific interviewing skills and strategies described in this text. The central tenet of this chapter is that interviewers must appreciate the importance a patient's beliefs have for his or her health-related behaviors and decisions. Thus, to understand their patients and provide effective care, skilled physicians must always strive to understand these beliefs.

THE CULTURE CONCEPT

Culture consists of the patterns of beliefs, values, understandings, and behaviors shared by an identifiable *group* of people. Because every individual is a member of numerous groups, everyone is a member of many cultures. Consider the following hypothetical person:

Mary Sanchez Smith is a 37-year-old woman of Mexican descent who was born and raised in El Paso, Texas, in a middle-class neighborhood. She is fluent in Spanish and English. A graduate of Baylor University College of Medicine, Mary is an associate professor of internal medicine at a major medical school. Mary is married to a physician of European-American descent, and she is the mother of two children. Raised a Catholic, Mary converted to a Protestant faith in college and is an active member of her congregation. Thus Mary is simultaneously a member of several different groups (ethnic, gender, class, occupation, religious, and family), each having its own particular set of values, beliefs, and behavioral expectations. Mary's perspective on life, her values and attitudes, and her actions all represent a unique blend or amalgam of these various cultures.

Culture should not be seen simply as a unified entity or "thing" that *determines* how a patient will behave. To think of culture as a thing that determines behavior is to risk acting on stereotypical beliefs about patients based on assumptions about the culture to which they belong. An important task for the skilled and culturally sensitive interviewer is to identify the beliefs, values, expectations, and behaviors that are probably influencing the way a patient perceives his or her health and well-being, and to determine how these cultural beliefs bear on the patient's responses to diagnostic and treatment recommendations. Culturally sensitive care "is a system that . . . is sensitive to intragroup variations in beliefs and behaviors, and avoids labeling and stereotyping."[2]

In a real sense, every medical encounter is a cross-cultural experience. As a result of physicians' training and enculturation into Western "biomedicine," they speak their own language and see disease and illness in a particular way. Colds have been transformed into "URIs" (upper respiratory infections). A "racing heart" in the vocabulary of a patient is translated as "tachycardia" in the lexicon of the physician. Practitioners of medicine rely on the senses of touch, sound, and sight in ways that are foreign to patients. Physicians rely on technologies that are unique to their professional culture and unfathomable to those who are not members of that culture. Mishler[3] has described the different perspectives that the voice of medicine and the voice of the life world bring with them to the medical encounter.

By being alert to the differences inherent in the perspectives of physicians and patients, the interviewer is taking the first step in providing culturally sensitive and, ultimately, culturally appropriate care. The second step in that process is to actively and systematically elicit the patient's perspective (his or her "explanatory model"). The third step involves exploring the implications of this perspective for the treatment to be provided.

IMPORTANCE OF UNDERSTANDING THE PATIENT'S "EXPLANATORY MODEL"

The physician-anthropologist Arthur Kleinman has been a pioneer in elucidating the importance of understanding patients' explanatory models of illness.[4] A patient's explanatory model consists of ideas about the nature and cause of the illness, notions about its seriousness and prognosis, expectations about how it should be evaluated and treated, and beliefs about how the individual affected should respond to the illness. It is on the basis of these explanatory models that patients make decisions about whether to consult the physician in the first place and, having made this decision, about whether to accept his or her explanations and advice. Because individuals construct explanatory models out of their unique experiences and the influence of various groups and cultures, it is not surprising that these models can be highly variable, even among individuals who are members of the same cultural groups. Furthermore, explanatory models vary in their content, coherency, and organization. Some explanatory models are highly structured and elaborate. Others are largely implicit, informal, and changeable.

Strategies for Eliciting Explanatory Models

Based on a wealth of clinical and research experience in the United States and China, Kleinman[4] has proposed a menu of questions that can be useful for eliciting a patient's explanatory model. These questions include the following:

- What do you call your problem? Does it have a particular name or label?
- What do you think is causing your problem?
- Why do you think it started when it did?
- How does this illness work? What is going on in your body?
- What kind of treatment do you think would be best for this problem?
- How has this problem affected your life and that of people around you?
- Is there anything in particular that you think needs to be done to figure out what is wrong?
- What worries you most about this problem or about its treatment?

It is not necessary to ask each of these questions of every patient. Rather, these questions are to be drawn upon selectively in an effort to understand the patient's concerns and to interpret the data that have been gathered. In some situations a question or two will quickly establish that the clinician and the patient are in substantial agreement about the problem, its meaning, and how it should be treated. In other situations, the physician may be surprised by the patient's responses and will need to spend more time and select more items from the menu to gain a fuller appreciation of the patient's beliefs and experience.

Medical students and physicians sometimes assume that necessary information on the patient's explanatory model will emerge spontaneously throughout the routine medical interviewing process. This is not the case. It is almost always necessary to actively and systematically elicit and explore the patient's perspective.[1]

The task of eliciting the patient's explanatory model is often more difficult than it may seem at first. The interviewer should realize that for a variety of reasons patients might be reluctant to give voice to their ideas. Some may feel embarrassed and self-conscious. Others may take it for granted that their views and the physician's are congruent. Still others may not want to bias the investigation.

The application of many of the skills discussed in this text to promote the development of rapport and to elicit accurate information will facilitate the disclosure of explanatory model data. In particular, it is important for the interviewer to approach the issue with genuine interest and nonjudgmental curiosity. He or she will also need to be persistent and flexible when phrasing questions. It is not uncommon for a patient to deny having any ideas at all (i.e., a personal explanatory model) about the nature of his or her problem when first asked. When this happens, the interviewer should ask again in a different way. The value of gentle persistence is illustrated by the following example of a family physician interacting with a patient who is concerned about menstrual irregularities and her inability to conceive a child. After a discussion of the patient's symptoms, the following exchange took place:

Physician: What do you think might be going on?
Patient: I don't know. I'm confused.
Physician: Confused? Well, is there anything that you've wondered about or been worried about?
Patient: (Following a brief pause) Tumors or something like that.
Physician: Tumors. That would be worrisome. Well, I'll be very careful about investigating what is going on so that we know exactly what we need to do. Is this something that your mother or sisters have talked to you about?
Patient: No. My mother is back in Colombia. It's just something that I've heard about.

This exchange took only seconds but provided the physician with important information. Had he not inquired about the patient's beliefs, he might not have learned so early in their relationship that she was concerned about cancer as well as her difficulties to conceive. Had he accepted the patient's first response—"I don't know, I'm confused"—he might not have known how best to allay the patient's fears and explain the rationale behind the diagnostic workup he wished to pursue. In this case persistence, flexibility, and genuine, nonjudgmental interest in the patient's perspective paid dividends for physician and patient alike.

Medical students and experienced practitioners often feel awkward about asking the patients for their ideas about what might be wrong with them, or about how the problem should be investigated and treated. It is not uncommon for a patient to say something such as the following:

Patient: I don't know what's wrong, that's why I came to see you!

When this happens, one or more of the following responses might help with the exploration of the patient's culturally mediated beliefs or worries:

Physician: I find that many of my patients have their own ideas or things they've heard about and it's helpful for me to know what they have been considering.

or

Is there something that you've worried about with these symptoms that you've been having?

or

Have you known anyone else with a problem like this? What did it turn out to be in that person's case?

or

Is there something that your (mother, wife, husband . . .) thinks is causing your problem and thinks we should check out?

CONTINUUM OF ILLNESS BELIEFS

When considering patients' explanatory models, it is helpful to think of a continuum of beliefs.[5] On one end are patients' explanatory models that are highly consistent with Western medicine's biomedical perspective. The midpoint consists of illness episodes in which a physician's biomedical perspective diverges from the patient's point of view. Examples of these midpoint divergences are the patient with a viral illness who is convinced he needs an antibiotic to treat the "infection" or the patient suffering from hypertension who feels that her condition is a stress-induced illness and that she only needs to take her medications when she feels acutely stressed. The other end of the continuum consists of explanatory models describing conditions that do not correspond at all with existing biomedical concepts. These are sometimes referred to as "folk illnesses" or "culture-bound syndromes" associated with membership in particular ethnic or national cultural groups. They are the conditions people often think of when considering issues of cultural sensitivity and culturally appropriate care. Examples of folk illness are *empacho,* a gastrointestinal ailment recognized by some Latino ethnic groups, and the Haitian illness *gaz,* or gas that can cause pain and discomfort in the head, shoulders, arms, or stomach. It is important to remember that not every member of an identifiable ethnic group adheres to a specific set of illness beliefs or behaviors. Often as much variation exists within cultural groups as between cultures.

The distinction between ideological and behavioral ethnicity may be useful for understanding and predicting the saliency of ethnic cultural traditions in patients' illness behaviors. An ideological ethnicity is one in which a person acknowledges and takes pride in his or her ethnic heritage without that heritage being a dominant factor influencing beliefs, attitudes, and daily behaviors. Behavioral ethnicity is another matter. The cultural roots of the behaviorally ethnic patient are likely to exert considerable influence over daily actions, beliefs, values, and responses to illness. The potential for a mismatch between the biomedical perspectives of the physician and patient is much greater in interactions with behaviorally ethnic patients. Pachter[2] lists several characteristics associated with "adherence to ethnocultural beliefs and behaviors," including the following:

1. Recent immigration to the host country
2. Residence in ethnic enclaves or neighborhoods
3. A preference for speaking in the native language
4. Formal education in the country of origin
5. Frequent return visits to the country of origin
6. Frequent contact with older, unacculturated persons from their native country

When the interview reveals that one or more of these patterns fits a patient, the physician should be alert to the possibility that the patient might not share the physician's biomedically rooted beliefs and understanding, especially since the United States is in the midst of a dramatic increase in the numbers of people immigrating from elsewhere in the world. Indeed, the current rate of immigration is rapidly approaching that of the period between 1901 and 1910, when close to 9 million people left their countries of origin for what they hoped would be a better life in the United States. The sharpest increases in the modern era have been in people from Asian and Pacific nations and people of Hispanic origin from various countries in Central and South America. By early in the next decade, people of Hispanic origin will represent the largest ethnic minority group in the United States. Every region of the United States has seen an increase in the number of immigrants from other countries.[5]

These demographic changes mark the increasing importance of physicians appreciating and attending to the cultural differences between patients and physicians that can affect medical care. Not only does this trend have significant implications for the prevalence of medically relevant behavioral ethnicity, it also raises issues about significant language barriers to effective medical communication when the physician does not understand the patient's native tongue.

WORKING WITH INTERPRETERS IN THE MEDICAL ENCOUNTER

Overcoming language barriers can be a difficult and often frustrating task for physician and patient alike. Effective interpretation in medical settings requires considerable skill on the part of both the interpreter and the physician. The interpreter's job is to accurately and clearly "describe and explain terms, ideas, and processes that lie outside of the linguistic system" of both the physician and the patient.[6] Effective medical interpreters do more than merely translate. They are also familiar with the ethnic culture and local community of the patient and are able not only to communicate the words spoken by the patient and the physician, but also to convey the "ideas, concerns, and rationales of each." As Hardt[7] notes, "Regardless of how the provider phrases a question or provides an answer, an effective interpreter is able to express the content of the message on the appropriate level of the patient's language."

Unfortunately, the task of interpreting for a patient who does not speak English often falls to anyone who happens to be available and conversant in both languages. This is often a family member, usually a child or friend. At other times, interpreting duties may be performed by a member of the hospital or doctor's office staff, regardless of the level of training and preparation to assume this important role. Use of nonprofessional interpreters should be avoided if possible because they have difficulty remaining neutral. Family members often have their own concerns and agendas because the illness affects them as much as it affects the patient. The patient may also be reluctant to divulge information that he or she does not want a family member or member of the community to know about. Hospital or office staff members drafted into that role by reasons of convenience may take editorial license in the translation process, based on their interest in conveying a particular image of the patient and the group to which they belong.[6]

Interpretation should be performed by a person who has been carefully selected and trained for this important and complicated task. Consider the simple example of translating a term like "allergy" or "allergic reactions." In many languages there is no one-to-one linguistic equivalent for the concept of allergy. A person who is untrained to make such translations would be hard pressed to do the job adequately.

Enhancing the Patient-Interpreter-Physician Interaction Before the Encounter

Before the actual interview, the physician should spend a couple of minutes reviewing the goals and objectives of the forthcoming visit with the interpreter. This can save time in the long run and can reduce the risk of misunderstandings. If the person serving as the translator has come with the patient, the interviewer should find out as much as possible about the relationship between the two. Physicians often must turn to a family member if an unrelated, professionally trained interpreter is not available. In such cases the clinician should attempt to find out that family member's own agenda and concerns before the interview begins. The physician should make it clear to the family member that full and accurate translation is the best and probably the only way to adequately address the concerns of both the translator and the patient.

The physician should convey the sense that he or she and the interpreter are partners in meeting the patient's needs. It can be useful to invite the interpreter to share his or her sense of the interaction and of the patient's story. Does the interpreter get the sense that the patient is anxious, frustrated, angry, or worried, or that the patient is holding back?

Whenever the physician is in a setting that involves caring for numbers of patients who are members of a specific ethnic culture, becoming familiar with health-related phrases or words in these patients' native language is advisable. Knowing the names commonly used to label illnesses, folk treatments, or folk healers will help the clinician track the interaction between the patient and the interpreter. This knowledge will also suggest avenues for further investigation and will convey to the patient that the doctor is interested in his or her beliefs and traditions. This can be an important aid to developing a rapport with the patient and can also facilitate the data-gathering and information-sharing functions of the interview.

During the Encounter

To the extent possible, the interviewer should arrange the seating in the examination room to allow for the physician, the patient, and the interpreter to have face-to-face contact. The patient should be addressed directly throughout the interview. The physician should avoid directing all of his or her questions and comments to the interpreter. Once a question has been asked or a comment has been made, the physician should signal the interpreter to commence with the translation. This helps regulate the pace and flow of information. When the patient is speaking, the physician's gaze should be directed at the patient. The physician needs to observe the patient carefully during the interpreter-patient exchanges, watching for nonverbal behaviors and cues. The physician will typically notice that the patient demonstrates emotional reactions (e.g., appears sad, smiles or laughs, changes the tone of his or her voice, or demonstrates any other behavior that strikes the interviewer as potentially relevant to the medical situation). In such instances the physician should ask the interpreter about these observations, especially if he or she cannot evaluate their significance based on the content of the interpretation.

Occasionally the physician will notice that something has probably been omitted in the translation. For example, after a lengthy exchange the interpreter may provide only a brief translation. In such cases the physician should gently remind the interpreter how important it is to get the full story and should request that nothing be left out. Problems of this sort are less likely to arise when working with a well-trained professional interpreter.

The clinician should check his or her understanding with the interpreter and invite the interpreter to offer corrections or alternative understandings. If the interviewer does not understand the interpretation, he or she should ask for clarification.

Guidelines for Language Use

The physician can do a number of things to make the interpreter's task more manageable. Questions should be brief and to the point. Similarly, when the physician is offering explanations or giving instructions, short sentences and frequent pauses will translate easier for the interpreter. Medical terminology and professional jargon should be avoided as much as possible because these terms may interfere with the interpreter's ability to translate accurately and efficiently. Idiomatic expressions or culture-bound metaphors should also be avoided. When translated literally, a statement like, "Let's make sure we are in the same ballpark" may produce little more than a puzzled stare from a patient who is unfamiliar with the expression.

Above all, when working with an interpreter, the physician needs to be patient. These encounters take more time, and the physician must try to avoid taking shortcuts out of a sense of time urgency.

Negotiating Culturally Sensitive Treatment Plans

After eliciting the patient's explanatory model, the physician is in a position to make judgments about the implications of that model for subsequent treatment and decision making. When the patient's explanatory model is close to that held by the physician, and when adherence to a particular model poses little risk of interfering with the patient's ability and willingness to follow treatment recommendations, providing information may be all that is required.

When adherence to a particular model or a strong belief in an ethnomedical system poses a risk for serious negative outcomes, a more "assertive" intervention is needed. However, such an intervention must be implemented in a respectful manner that preserves the relationship and offers the potential of developing a partnership with the patient. The following examples are illustrative:

Case 1: *Mrs. Jones is a 57-year-old woman who has hypertension. Her family history is significant for high blood pressure and premature death caused by heart disease. Mrs. Jones has a BA in business administration and works full-time as office manager for a small law firm. She is pleasant and cooperative and always keeps her appointments with her doctor. A little more than a year after Mrs. Jones was placed on medications, her blood pressure is still not well controlled. Suspecting that Mrs. Jones may not be taking her medications as prescribed, her physician decides to spend more time inquiring about how she takes her medications and about her understanding of hypertension.*

This discussion led to the discovery that Mrs. Jones thinks of hypertension as a stress-related disorder ("hyper-tension"). She also believes she can tell when her blood pressure is up by the presence of tension headaches. Mrs. Jones indicates that when she feels acutely stressed or experiences a headache, she feels she needs to be taking her medication. However, when she is not feeling particularly stressed and is not having headaches, she believes that her blood pressure is not a problem and does not require treatment. Armed with this information, the physician was able to explain that hypertension is a condition that has multiple causes and that one's blood pressure can be persistently high even in the absence of perceptible stress. He was also able to explain that hypertension does not always produce symptoms that can be reliably linked to blood pressure elevations. He went on to propose that Mrs. Jones take her medications consistently over the next 6 weeks, regardless of whether she felt stressed or experienced tension headaches, and that she return following this trial period to see how her blood pressure was doing. Mrs. Jones agreed to this, and on her return visit 6 weeks later her blood pressure was in the normal range.

Case 2: *Mrs. Gonzalez is a young Puerto Rican woman who lives in a large urban center in the northeastern United States. She arrives at the clinic in obvious distress about her 7-month-old son, who has been treated for the past 3 months for asthma by a pediatrician who does not speak Spanish. Although Mrs. Gonzalez speaks some English, she is most comfortable using her native Spanish. At this visit the pediatrician decided to employ the assistance of a trained Spanish-language interpreter who herself is a native of Puerto Rico. The patient admitted to the interpreter that she did not believe the medications prescribed by the* *physician at the last visit were helping her child. She also disclosed that her parents felt that the child's illness was most likely the result of evil spirits and that she should take him to an Espiritista for proper treatment.*

Mrs. Gonzalez was at a loss. On the one hand, she was very worried about her baby and wondered if her parents might be right about what was causing his problem. On the other hand, she had developed a good relationship with her pediatrician and she did not wish to offend him. On learning about Mrs. Gonzalez's concerns, the doctor, through the interpreter, reached an agreement that she would continue giving her baby the medicines he had prescribed, and that she would also consult the Espiritista. Following this consultation, Mrs. Gonzalez agreed to return to the clinic and tell the doctor about the Espiritista's recommendations. That way, he could assess whether folk treatment posed any kind of risks to the baby. If it did not, the pediatrician was happy to have Mrs. Gonzalez employ both Western and folk medical traditions in the care of her child. Mrs. Gonzalez left the encounter reassured that she could trust her doctor to be open and respectful of her beliefs, willing to continue the treatments he prescribed, and relieved that she could also consult with a healer valued in her ethnic cultural community.

Although the content of these two cases varies considerably, the strategies employed by the physicians are similar. In each, the physician made an effort to elicit and to understand the patient's beliefs. Rather than dismissing the explanatory models and beliefs of the patient and simply trying to convince the patient to accept the physician's biomedical perspective, each entered into a partnership. In the case of Mrs. Jones, the physician was able to negotiate a trial period in which she would take her medications regardless of how she was feeling. He did not simply negate her belief that she could tell when her blood pressure was elevated, but suggested an alternative understanding of her illness and a way for her to test this alternative.

In the case of Mrs. Gonzalez, the physician worked out a compromise that enabled her to visit a folk healer without abandoning the biomedical care that he was providing. By having Mrs. Gonzalez return to the clinic and report the treatment proposed by the *Espiritista,* he was also in a position to assess whether that treatment might be harmful to the baby. If the latter turned out to be the case, he would have to negotiate another compromise with the patient. In this case the services of the trained Puerto Rican interpreter would no doubt come in handy.

Fortunately, most folk remedies and treatments have been found to be relatively safe. For those that are not, it is often possible to work with the folk practitioner to find alternatives that do not produce harmful side effects. In this case the physician not only enters into partnership with the patient, but also sends a clear message of respect and conveys a willingness to be supportive.

CONCLUSION

To be sure, cross-cultural medical encounters pose unique challenges, but they also provide unique opportunities to learn from patients. The mnemonic ***LEARN*** may help medical students and physicians elicit and understand patients' explanatory models and cultural beliefs.[8]

1. ***L****isten* with sympathy and understanding to the patient's beliefs and concerns.
2. ***E****xplain* your own perceptions, understandings, and beliefs.
3. ***A****cknowledge* and explore differences and similarities in beliefs.
4. ***R****ecommend* treatment.
5. ***N****egotiate* agreement.

Culturally sensitive interviewing first requires mastery of the basic skills discussed in this text, integrated with the appreciation that all medical encounters, to varying degrees, involve differences in cultural beliefs and understandings. Medical students and physicians who develop these skills will be in an excellent position to understand each of their patients as unique individual products of many different cultural influences. This understanding will contribute directly to improved medical care. It will facilitate the accurate and efficient elicitation of data and will better enable the physician to provide information to the patient in a manner that will promote the patient's understanding and adherence to treatment recommendations. Most important, perhaps, it will lead to the development of the kinds of relationships that motivated the physician to become a healer in the first place.

REFERENCES

1. Johnson TM, Hardt EJ, Kleinman A: Cultural factors in the medical interview. In Lipkin M Jr, Putnam SM, Lazare A, editors: *The medical interview: clinical care, education, and research*, New York, 1995, Springer-Verlag.
2. Pachter LM: Culture and clinical care: folk illness beliefs and behaviors and their implications for health care delivery, *JAMA* 271(9):690-694, 1994.
3. Mishler EG: *The discourse of medicine: dialectics of medical interviews*, Norwood, NJ, 1984, Ablex.
4. Kleinman A: *Patients and healers in the context of culture: an exploration of the borderland between anthropology, medicine, and psychiatry*, Berkeley, 1980, University of California Press.
5. Buchwald D, Caralis P, Gany F, et al: Caring for patients in a multicultural society, *Patient Care* 28(11):105-123, 1994.

6. Putsch RW: Cross-cultural communication: the special case of interpreters in health care, *JAMA* 254(23):3344-3348, 1985.
7. Hardt EJ: Discussion leader's guide: the bilingual medical interview I and the bilingual medical interview II: the geriatric interview, Boston, Boston Department of Health and Hospitals.
8. South-Paul JE: Negotiation with patients. In Mengle MB, Fields SA, editors: *Introduction to clinical skills: a patient-centered textbook,* New York, 1997, Plenum Medical Book.

CHAPTER

20 Family Interviewing

Kathy Cole-Kelly
Thomas L. Campbell

THE ROLE OF THE FAMILY IN HEALTH CARE

Interviewing patients' families is an important skill for all physicians. Families are the primary context within which most health problems and illnesses occur. Research results have demonstrated that the family has a powerful influence on health and illness.[1] Most health beliefs and behaviors (e.g., smoking, diet, and exercise) are developed and maintained within the family.[2] Marital and family relationships have as powerful an impact on health outcomes as biologic factors.[3] Family interventions have been shown to improve health outcomes for a variety of health problems.[4]

Family members, not health professionals, are the primary health care providers for most patients. Outside the hospital, health care professionals give advice and suggestions for the acute and chronic illness, but the actual care is usually provided by the patient (self-care) and family members. With the aging of the population comes a significant increase in the prevalence of chronic illness and disability and a rise in family caregiving. For example, most patients with Alzheimer's disease are cared for at home by family members.

Unfortunately, families are often neglected in health care. Our culture focuses on the individual and emphasizes autonomy over connectedness. The effect of serious illness on other family members is often ignored. Recently, family-centered models that actively involve parents and siblings in the child's care have been developed for hospitals and outpatient clinics from within the specialty of pediatrics. Family practice developed around the concept of caring for the entire family and treating the family as the patient. However, in most of the medical community, the family is rarely engaged as an active partner in health care. The ability to work effectively with families and to use them as a resource in patient care is an essential skill for all physicians, regardless of specialty.

SITUATIONS IN WHICH FAMILY MEMBERS ARE OFTEN PRESENT

Although at times arranging or convening a family meeting to discuss health issues is important, the most frequent opportunities for interviewing family members are the times they accompany the patient to the hospital or physician's office. Family members are usually the ones who bring a patient to the hospital, and they can serve as valuable informants about the patient's health problem. Unfortunately, family members are usually excluded from the emergency room, where they could have served as informants. During outpatient visits it can be useful to inquire whether family members are in the waiting room and to include them in the initial interview.

With more liberal visiting hours in hospitals, family members are often at the bedside of patients. Family members may be present during morning rounds or the initial hospital evaluation. Rather than routinely requesting that the family member leave during the evaluation, finding out about the family member and the role the patient would like the person to take is helpful. For example, most spouses would like to remain with the patient during medical interviews and examinations (except pelvic and rectal examinations). They often feel better informed about their spouse's condition and treatment and reassured by the care that the spouse is receiving. Studies have shown that even during distressing procedures such as cardiopulmonary resuscitation, family members would prefer to observe what is happening.[5]

In the outpatient setting, family members are often present in several situations. During pregnancy care the father of the baby frequently attends a prenatal visit and should be actively involved in the interview. Involving fathers in pregnancy and infant care can help increase the father's sense of connection and involvement with both the pregnancy and the infant. Thus involvement can have beneficial effects for the infant and the entire family. During well- and ill-child visits, one and sometimes both parents routinely accompany the child. After assessing the developmental level of the child, the clinician can decide how to balance the interview and talk with both the child and the parent. For infants and very young children the entire interview is with the parent(s). When a parent accompanies an adolescent to a medical visit, the physician must decide when to meet separately with the adolescent and how much to involve the parent.

An increasingly common situation occurs when an elderly patient is brought in by a family member who may serve as the primary family caregiver. This is usually an adult child, often a daughter, or the patient's spouse. Deciding how to involve the family caregiver in the interview is parallel to interviewing parents and children. The goal is to include the patient as much as possible, depending on the patient's cognitive abilities. For severely demented patients the interview is mostly with the family caregiver.

The Three Functions of Family Interviewing

The principles of interviewing an individual patient also apply to interviewing families, but there are additional complexities. The physician must engage and talk with at least one additional person, and the opportunity exists for interaction between the patient and family members. In general, the physician must be more active and establish clear leadership in a family interview. This may be as simple as being certain that each participant's voice is heard ("Mrs. Jones, we haven't heard from you about your concerns about your husband's illness. Can you share those?") or acting as a "traffic cop" with a large and vocal family ("Jim, I know that you have some ideas about your mother's care, but I'd like to let your sister finish talking before we hear from you.") The next sections of the chapter contain a discussion of how the three functions of interviewing can be applied systematically to interviewing families.

FUNCTION 1: BUILDING THE RELATIONSHIP

When working with families, establishing rapport and developing a relationship is known as *joining*. An essential component of joining is making some positive contact with each person present so that each feels valued and connected enough to the physician to participate in the interview. Family members have often been excluded from health care discussions and decisions, even when they are present. They may not expect to be included in the interview or to be asked to participate in decision making. By making contact with each person, the physician is making it clear that everyone is encouraged to participate in the interview.

There are several other important reasons for joining with family members at the beginning of the interview. The clinician often has an established relationship with the patient but not with other family members. The family member may feel left out or that his or her role is merely that of an observer. One common example of this occurs during hospital rounds when there is a family member by the bedside. The usual approach is either to ask family members to leave during the interview or to ignore them. This approach is not respectful of families and fails to use the family as a resource. This alternative approach is suggested:

1. After greeting the patient, greet and shake hand with the family member and introduce yourself.

Physician: Good morning, Mrs. Janeway (the patient). (Turn to family member and shake hands.) Hello, I'm Frank Medcoci. I'm the medical student on the team taking care of Mrs. Janeway.

Usually family members will introduce themselves and state their relationship to the patient.

> **Family member:** Nice to meet you. I'm Mrs. Janeway's daughter, Mary.

It is helpful to learn what the family member's relationship is to the patient because the physician may deal differently with a son, daughter, or spouse than with a nephew or someone who is not a family member. If the family member does not provide this information, you can usually obtain it by asking, "And you are?" or, "And how are you related to Mrs. Janeway?"

2. Obtain the patient's permission to talk with the family member who is present. This can usually be done quickly and easily.

> **Physician:** Mrs. Janeway, before I ask you about how your night went, I'd like to talk with your relative (or husband, daughter, etc.) for a minute. Would that be okay with you?

Asking for the patient's permission, which is rarely denied or even questioned, is respectful to the patient and reassures the patient that the physician will be spending time talking with the patient as well.

3. Involve the family member in the interview from the beginning by asking a question such as the following:

> **Physician:** How do you feel your mother (or Mrs. Janeway) is doing?

This question involves the daughter in the interview and communicates that the physician is interested in her viewpoint. It can also provide some important medical information. For example:

> **Family member:** She looks okay now, but earlier this morning she threw up a bunch of blood.

A similar situation involving a family member's presence often occurs when fathers attend prenatal visits. Fathers commonly feel marginalized during a pregnancy and may view themselves as merely observers, not as active participants and partners. They may sit in the corner of the examination room and remain silent and uninvolved if not invited to participate. It is important to greet the father of the baby at the beginning of the interview and to recognize his role.

> **Physician:** Hi, I'm Dr. Campbell (shaking hands). You are?
> **Father:** Darrell.

Physician: It's very nice to meet you, Darrell. I'm really glad that you came in with your partner (or wife or fiancée). I think it is really important for a dad to be involved in the pregnancy and delivery. You are welcome to any of these visits. Can you tell me a little about yourself?

An important step in joining is communicating respect for the family member and his or her opinions. For many men, this can be done by inquiring about their job and showing interest in their work:

Physician: What kind of work do you do, Darrell?

If the father is unemployed, the physician can discuss the challenges of looking for work. This step usually takes only a minute or two, but strongly communicates an interest in that person's life. As with Mrs. Janeway's daughter, the physician could then ask Darrell:

Physician: How do you think your girlfriend has been doing during the pregnancy?

Later in the pregnancy, it would be important to inquire about how he would like to be involved in the labor and delivery.

Special issues are involved when children are present during the interview. Children are often expected to be seen and not heard in a clinical encounter involving their parent or another family member. However, they may have many questions or misconceptions about the family member's illness.

Jim and Betsy Werner brought their 9-year-old daughter Rachel with them to Betsy's appointment with her oncologist. After discussing the next stage of treatment for Betsy's breast cancer, the oncologist asked Rachel if she had any questions. She asked, "Can I catch breast cancer from my mother?"

Children are more likely to participate in the interview and ask questions if the physician takes just a few moments to connect with them and make them feel important. With small children, a quick comment such as, "Gee, I like your sweatshirt," or, "I wish I had cool barrettes like those" can be enough to signal that the physician is interested in them. With older children and adolescents, a respectful "Hello," "Glad to meet you," and "If you have any questions, I hope you will feel free to ask them" can give them the message that the physician is pleased to have them there, while giving them enough space not to feel pressured.

WHEN THERE IS CONFLICT IN THE FAMILY

Establishing a positive relationship with family members is particularly important and more challenging when there is conflict in the family. In these cases the family member will usually assume that the physician has taken the side of the patient in the conflict. In situations of conflict the physician must take extra steps to join with the family members and establish his or her neutrality. The goal is to develop an alliance with each family member and the patient without taking sides in the conflict. An exception to this goal is a situation in which family violence threatens one person's physical safety. Dealing with family conflict and violence is discussed in more detail later in the chapter.

In addition to establishing rapport and building a relationship through verbal communication, the physician can make use of nonverbal strategies to enhance the relationship with the patient and family members. Just as it is important to be sure that the physician and an individual patient are in a comfortable sitting position and at eye level with each other, so is it important that other family members are sitting or standing (if the room doesn't have enough chairs) near enough that they can hear what is being said and can be easily seen by the physician. This proximity to voice and face will help the physician make eye contact with each person in the room.

On entering the room and seeing that one family member is sitting far from the physician or is isolated from other family members, the physician can gently motion that person to come closer. This will enhance everyone's sense of being included in the patient visit and of being an important part of the encounter. If one family member seems to be sitting or standing particularly far from the center of the clinical action, the physician might want to take the time to encourage the person to come closer to the action in the room. Otherwise, the family member taking a more distant position might be harder to build a relationship with during the encounter. Similarly, one family member might dominate both the verbal and nonverbal space in the encounter, making it difficult for the other family members to have as much involvement in the action with the patient or physician.

To encourage a relationship with the quieter members and discourage domination by louder members, the physician can use both verbal and nonverbal cues to ensure a connection with all the family members present. For example:

Family member: I'm so concerned about my mother. She has been in the hospital far too often. I don't think the doctors are doing much here. I am really not at all . . .

Physician: Ms. Jones, I think I have a good understanding of what your concerns are and I want to respond to them, but I'd first like to hear from your brother, Mr. Norton. Mr. Norton, this is the first time I've met you and I'm wondering what your perspective is on your mother's condition. I'd like to hear your opinion. Maybe you could move your chair in a little closer so I can hear you better

FUNCTION 2: GATHERING INFORMATION FROM THE PATIENT AND FAMILY

As stated initially, family members are an invaluable resource to the physician. A family-sensitive interviewer sees the presence of other family members as the opportunity for gathering important information about the patient and his or her health care context. The physician can gather information about the patient's and family's understanding of the illness, important health history information, current stressors affecting the patient, and potential resources to help the patient's care. In addition, the physician can gather information from the family about who is currently involved in the patient's care. This can be important for the physician to know when making treatment plans.

The initial step in gathering this information has been accomplished by the first function of interviewing: joining and relationship building. Without this step, family members will not appreciate their importance in the medical interview. Part of this initial joining and relationship building includes finding out exactly who is in the room and how each person is related to the patient. Once this has been accomplished and contact has been made with each person in the room, the physician can begin to gather information from the family.

The physician's goal is usually to gather information that helps with diagnosis or treatment planning. The family members may have their own agendas, which could be the reason they have come with the patient to the visit. Thus it is helpful to elicit the reason that each family member has come to the visit.

Physician: Hi, I'm Dr. White. I don't believe I've met you before. (joining)

Family member: Oh, I'm Joey's father. I'm out of town a lot but was worried when I heard he was in the hospital, and my mother-in-law let me know he was here.

Physician: Great of you to come. Are there any questions I can answer for you? I'd like to hear your perspective on how Joey manages his diabetes. (gathering the information)

Family member: Well, yes, I'm sort of worried about Joey's care because his mother has been so preoccupied with our new baby. I'm wondering if something else can be done so he doesn't keep ending up in the hospital.

By seeing the father as a resource, the physician gathers information in this brief interaction about the relationship to the child, a beginning hint of his involvement (out of town a lot), and his major concern (wife being overwhelmed and thus less attentive to Joey's diabetes).

The physician faces a more delicate challenge when gathering information about an adolescent patient. Issues of confidentiality are heightened during adolescence. Adolescents' attitudes span a continuum from determined to retain a strong sense of independence to comfortable with parents involved in both their health care and the interview. This has implications for the way the physician conducts the family interview. The physician first needs to inquire about the adolescent's comfort with questions being asked in the presence of his or her parents. Once this has been established, the physician can proceed by gathering information, either separately or with the family and adolescent together.

In addition to the verbal information the physician can gather from the family members present in the room, he or she can also gather important information through observations of where people sit and how they participate in the interview. Where family members sit in the examination room often tells the clinician something about relationships and roles in the family. For instance, how close a couple sits together is often a measure of their emotional closeness. A family member who sits across the examination room in the corner may reveal a sense of being an observer or a nonparticipant in the patient's care.

In addition to observing where family members place themselves relative to the patient in the room, noting where the family members sit or stand relative to the physician can be revealing. A family member's taking the chair closest to the physician often indicates that the family member feels he or she is or should be in charge of the patient's care. This can give the physician information about differing levels of involvement in the patient's care. This observation could be useful information, triggering questions about relationships between members of the family and the patient.

Noting where patients and family members sit when the physician enters an examination or hospital room is important; however, this seating arrangement should not necessarily be accepted as the structure for conducting the interview. Just as the physician asks the patient to sit or lie on the examination table to facilitate the physical examination, so should the physician arrange chairs and family members to facilitate involvement of all family members in the interview. This might include asking a shy family member to pull up a chair next to the patient, or having the child sitting on the examination table move to the chair next to the physician, with the parent next to the child. By rearranging where the patient and family members are sitting, the physician is also making a statement about what roles he or she would like them to play, that is, "who the patient is" (sitting next to the physician) and how the accompanying family members should participate. This is analogous to asking the passive patient who sits on the examination table waiting to be examined to sit next to the physician and assume a more participatory role.

> Mary McCarthy is 11 years old and has come into the hospital because of an exacerbation of her asthma. In the room are her mother Susan, her father Bill, and her brother Toby. Mary and her dad are sitting on the bed (or examination table), and Mom is sitting as far away as possible from them both.
>
> **Physician:** Susan, why don't you come closer to us so I have you all in a single range of vision. That's great. Now, tell me what you noticed about Mary last night before you brought her into the hospital.

Although there are significant advantages to having the family as a resource for gathering information about the patient and the context of care, the physician's fear of losing control of the interview can be a compelling disincentive. On walking into a roomful of family members, the physician may naturally feel overwhelmed and think it would be easier to interview the patient alone. However, several family-interviewing strategies can help the physician feel that he or she is able to gather information without relinquishing total control.

1. The physician can explain at the beginning that he or she is interested in each person's perspective and will be sure to hear each one.
2. If one person begins to dominate the interview, the physician should think of himself or herself as a benevolent traffic cop, putting up a hand to indicate time is up and interrupting the family member by saying something like the following:

> **Physician:** Mr. Goodman, I'd like to hear more from you, but I want to be sure to hear your wife and daughter's perspective. Then, if there's time, I'll get back to you.

3. In case a child begins to interrupt too much, the physician should make sure there are some toys in the office. The physician can also have the child sit near him or her, so that the physician may place a hand on the child's shoulder or leg and signal the child to "hush" if necessary.
4. The physician should avoid questions that might make family members feel blamed or create divisiveness between family members. In the course of gathering information about the patient's illness or treatment, discrepancies in family members' beliefs or approaches inevitably surface. It is important to avoid asking questions that could pit one family member against another.

Reframing information questions as queries that the physician would like clarified elicits the desired information while minimizing the potential for interpersonal explosions.

> **Physician:** It seems that you and your mother had different approaches to the feeding of the baby. Can you help me understand how that worked? (Special considerations for handling conflict or intense emotional responses during the family interview are discussed in the "Special Circumstances" section.)

FUNCTION 3: FAMILY EDUCATION, NEGOTIATION, AND MOTIVATION

All of the principles for education, negotiation, and motivation with an individual also apply to family members, with two important considerations. First, when delivering information to more than one person, it is important to recognize that each person is likely to have different knowledge, beliefs, and expectations about the medical problem and the prognosis and treatment. This must be taken into account when working with families. Second, family members can be an enormous resource in motivating patients to adhere to medical treatments or to change unhealthy behaviors. This family resource should be used to benefit the patient.

Delivering Information

One of the most common and important reasons for bringing families together and convening a family meeting is to deliver important medical information to the patient and his or her family. This often involves the delivery of bad news, such as the diagnosis of cancer or other life- threatening illness or a poor prognosis. For several reasons, patients should be encouraged to have family members with them when bad news will be given. First, the family members can be an important source of support for the patient during this stressful time. Second, patients often misunderstand information when the content is highly emotional. For example, a patient may interpret cancer as a death sentence even when the physician explains that the cancer is curable. The family members who are present can help correct these misconceptions. Third, family members often receive misinformation when it is relayed secondhand by the patient. In the case above, the patient might tell his family that he has terminal cancer. Physicians often receive phone calls from family members who did not receive the information directly. Delivering bad news with family members present allows the physician to see how the family reacts and will cope with the problem. The physician can learn how supportive or emotionally expressive the family will be.

Before providing information to family members, it is important to assess their current level of understanding, their beliefs, and their concerns, just as it is with individual patients. Knowing their baseline level of knowledge allows the physician to tailor the information that is provided and correct any misunderstandings. Understanding family members' fears can facilitate appropriate reassurances. If the physician initially takes the time to elicit the family's knowledge, beliefs, and concerns, the rest of the interview will be more efficient and effective.

Dr. C. is meeting with Mrs. Goldman and her family after she has been admitted with an exacerbation of her chronic obstructive lung disease.

Physician: I want to update you on your mother's medical condition, but before I do that, I'd like to know what your understanding of your mother's condition is.

Son: (provides description)

Physician: That's a very accurate description of what is going on with your mother. I want to come back to that, but first I want to know what others understand about what has happened.

One of Mrs. Goldman's daughters believes that her mother's breathing is made worse by the air conditioning in her apartment and that she needs to get more fresh air. Before correcting this misunderstanding, the physician elicits other beliefs and concerns about the patient's health. He then gives a brief summary of her condition, addressing each of the family members' concerns and beliefs.

In general, medical information should be provided to family members with the patient present and with his or her permission. Most patients want their family members to be informed about their medical conditions, but consent must be obtained.

Physician: I'd like to inform your family about your medical condition. Is there anything that you don't want me to share with them?

The patient may not want to have some sensitive information discussed with certain family members. The patient should be present during these family conferences whenever possible. This prevents misinformation or secrets from developing. In the hospital or nursing home, this means meeting with the family at the bedside. The family members may desire not to "burden" the patient with issues concerning prognosis or treatment plans. At an extreme, family members may not want the patient to receive the diagnosis of a terminal condition, believing, "It will just upset him too much" or, "If she finds out, she'll just give up." These efforts to protect the patient should be avoided because they lead to secrecy and a breakdown in communication.

> ***The Matthews family wanted to meet separately with Dr. K., their father's physician, and with the hospital social worker to decide on nursing home placement after Mr. Matthews's stroke. They knew that their father would be upset if he knew what they were talking about.***
>
> ***Dr. K. insisted that they all meet together, since they were talking about Mr. Matthews's future. The patient was upset at first when he learned about their proposal. However, as he heard family members express their love and concern for him and their fear that they could not care for him at home, he began to accept the idea of placement in a nursing home.***

Using the Family as a Resource in Motivating Patients to Change

Family members play an important role in developing and maintaining health behaviors. They can be a valuable resource in helping patients to adhere to medical treatments and change unhealthy behaviors. Almost every important health behavior is a family activity or is strongly influenced by the family. These behaviors are risk factors and tend to cluster within families, since family members tend to have similar diets, physical activities, and use of substances (e.g., tobacco, alcohol, and illicit drugs).[2] Parents' health-related behaviors strongly influence whether a child or adolescent will adopt a healthy behavior. In a Gallup survey of health-related behaviors, most adults reported that their spouse or partner was more likely to influence their health habits than anyone else, including their family doctor.

Support from family members has been associated with successful smoking cessation, weight loss, participation in exercise programs, and compliance with medical treatments. Family interventions have been successful in the treatment of cardiac risk factors, obesity, and compliance with hypertension treatment.[4] In one large study, providing family support to help with compliance with blood pressure medication resulted in improved compliance, reduced blood pressure, and a 50% reduction in cardiac mortality.[6] Based on this and similar compliance research, the National Heart, Lung and Blood Institute recommends that physicians use the following as one of three basic strategies for increasing adherence with antihypertensive regimens:

> Enhance support from family members. Identifying and involving one influential person, preferably someone living with the patient, who can provide encouragement helps support the behavior change and, if necessary, reminds the patient about the specifics of the regimen.[7]

Whether in the hospital or outpatient setting, the family can be used as a resource in the treatment plan anytime that a family member is present. The goal is to negotiate a treatment plan not just with the patient, but with the family as well. This is particularly important when the plan will have an effect on the family or must be carried out by family members. For example, it makes little sense to counsel most middle-aged men about low-fat diets without including their wives, who are usually responsible for the menu and cooking.

During an office visit the physician can help the patient negotiate with family members how they can be helpful to the patient in making behavioral changes. Consider the following dialogue:

Physician: So Jim, how do you think Karen (his wife) could help you remember to take your blood pressure medication?

Patient: Well, for one thing, it doesn't help when she nags me about it.

Physician: Okay, scratch that off the list. What could she do to help you?

Patient: Maybe if she put my pills out on the breakfast table, it would help me to remember.

Physician: All right, that sounds pretty simple. Karen, do you think you could do that?

Wife: Sure.

Physician: What else could she do? . . . (additional negotiations)

Physician: Jim, what should Karen do if she notices that you have forgotten to take your medication?

Patient: Just forget about it and don't nag me about taking them.

Physician: Karen, are you okay with that?

Wife: I guess so.

The goal of these sessions is to help couples and families come up with specific helpful and supportive interventions that are acceptable to the patient and the family. Marital or family conflicts or dysfunction can sometimes interfere with this process. One family member may sabotage the patient's attempts at changing unhealthy behaviors. It may be necessary in such cases to refer the family to a family therapist who can help with underlying family issues.

SPECIAL CIRCUMSTANCES WHEN INTERVIEWING FAMILIES

Interviewing families can present special challenges or circumstances that are not usually seen when interviewing individuals. This section discusses a few of the more common and important circumstances and issues that can occur when interviewing families.

When to Convene the Family

Although family members often accompany the patient to the hospital and outpatient appointment, sometimes inviting family members to a meeting or session to discuss medical issues is helpful. Research results have demonstrated that patients and families desire family conferences or meetings and request them for serious medical and psychosocial problems.[8] Although the physician should convene the family whenever he or she feels it might be helpful for the patient or family, there are four situations in which a routine family conference should be considered:

1. **Hospitalization:** It is helpful to meet with the family shortly after admission to explain the patient's condition and treatment and before discharge to discuss the family's role in outpatient care.
2. **Prenatal and well-child care:** Both parents should be invited and included in all prenatal and well-child visits.
3. **Death and dying:** It is important to meet with the family at the time of a terminal diagnosis, during the dying phase, and after death.
4. **Diagnosis of a serious chronic illness:** Anytime that a serious illness is diagnosed, involving the family can be helpful.

Family members will usually attend a family conference when invited by the physician, if the physician is positive and direct about the need to meet with the family, emphasizes the importance of the family in caring for the patient, and stresses the benefits of a family meeting to the patient and family.

Avoiding Taking Sides or Triangulation

A physician seeing multiple family members needs to learn to avoid becoming triangulated—being pulled into an alliance with one family member at the exclusion of another. The physician can be pulled unwittingly into unresolved conflicts between family members. In the case of an ill child, one parent may try to form an alliance with the physician that excludes the other parent. Or, a wife can try to get the physician on her side, hoping that the physician's alliance will bolster her position against her husband. To avoid being caught in the middle of a triangle, the physician needs to be facile at reassuring each member of the family that the physician is there to hear each person's story but not to take sides. Furthermore, the physician can assert that it will not be helpful to the family if the physician is pulled into an alliance with one member at the exclusion of another. The physician can emphasize the importance of everyone's working together as the most beneficial way to enhance the health care of the patient.

When the Customer Is Not the Patient

The customer is the person who desires a service and is not always the patient. Sometimes a family member may want some medical service or intervention for another family member. An obvious example is when a mother (customer) brings her young child (patient) in for treatment of a medical problem. A common but subtler case occurs when a middle-aged man is sent for a checkup by his wife because she is worried that he is not taking care of his health. Unless the physician inquires closely, the man may say that he is there for a checkup and that everything is fine.

When the patient is not the customer, it is helpful to talk directly with the customer to find out what the concerns or requests are. The wife of the middle-aged man might report that he has been having chest pains when they go for walks, but that he is reluctant to do anything about it. In some cases it may be helpful or even necessary to have the customer and patient in the examination room together. Consider the following phone call:

Patient: Dr. C., you are seeing my husband this afternoon and I wish that you would talk to him about his drinking. Recently, he has been getting drunk once or twice a week.

Physician: Mrs. James, I hear your concern about your husband's health. I'd like you to come in with your husband later today so we can talk about your concerns. I think he needs to hear this directly from you.

Recognizing when the customer is not the patient and communicating directly with the customer can help the physician from becoming triangulated or caught in family conflicts.

Dealing with Strong Affect During the Family Interview

The potential for family members to become very emotional is heightened when dealing with a critical life event such as a diagnosis of a serious illness (e.g., a newborn with cystic fibrosis or a middle-aged woman with breast cancer), a difficult decision (e.g., nursing home placement), and uncertainty (the course of the illness—for example, how long someone with chronic obstructive pulmonary disease has to live). When family members are offering their opinions about these difficult issues, one or many family members may have intense emotional feelings in response to the medical situation. Sadness and anger are the two most commonly expressed emotions when family members are confronting difficult medical situations.

The principles for dealing with strong affect in families are the same as those used when interviewing a single patient. In families, however, expressed feelings often trigger strong emotions in other family members and may intensify the affect.

When the physician is delivering bad news or discussing serious health problems, family members commonly express sorrow or grief. This can be beneficial for family members because it allows them to share their feelings and obtain support from one another. Often it can be helpful to shift the interview to an affective level and encourage family members to share their feelings with a question such as, "How are you all feeling about this?" In response to such a question, one family member may start sharing his or her emotional reactions, which may trigger another to start crying. The challenge for the physician is to refrain from intervening or interfering with this process. Many physicians treat tears like blood and try to stop any crying, usually because it makes the physician uncomfortable.

A few approaches by the physician can help during intense and sometimes stormy moments:

1. The physician should have tissues available to give the family members. Often it can be nice to hand the box to one member and ask him or her to give it to the emotional member.
2. The physician should be patient during this period and remember that it is better for the emotions to be expressed in the physician's presence. The physician and the other family members can be a witness to the feelings of the one member and can provide reassurance.

When anger is expressed by one member about a health outcome, it is important for the physician to listen, to reflect that he or she has heard how angry the patient or family member is, and to ask if others share that feeling. It can be valuable for the family members to experience their anger being heard. However, the physician should also feel confident about maintaining control of the situation during this time. When one family member is expressing frustration and anger for a few minutes, the physician and other family members should patiently listen; however, the physician may ask the family member to lower his or her voice while expressing the feeling. After hearing a few angry sentences, the physician can turn to the rest of the family members to ask if anyone would like to briefly add to the information being offered.

Family Member: (in a loud angry tone) I just don't understand why no one told us before about my wife's illness. I mean, I've been asking for someone to help us with her and I feel that everyone just keeps beating around the bush.

Physician: Mr. Platt, I understand your anger and frustration. These are difficult situations to predict, and I know it is hard to watch your spouse in this condition.

Family Member: Yes, but you and your staff just seem to. . . .

Physician: Mr. Platt, I'm going to interrupt you and give your son and daughter a chance to speak. Brenda (adult daughter) *or* Jon (adult son), do you share your father's frustration?

Listening to one member express frustration may trigger another family member to echo the feeling. Often families have a family member who takes the role of peacemaker and quiets the intense emotion in the room without intervention from the physician. However, if the anger is starting to intensify, the physician needs to interrupt as the physician above did and turn to another family member.

In addition to the expression of anger by various family members toward the health care system or the uncertainty of the situation, having multiple family members in one room increases the risk of conflict between family members. The intensity of the situation with a loved one can mobilize the family members' unresolved feelings of resentment or irritation toward one another. Sometimes the hospital is the first setting in which many of these members have gathered together in a long time. If sparks begin to fly between family members, it is important to provide them with a safe, controlled atmosphere. The physician needs to assert a sense of control by saying something like the following:

Physician: I think this is not the time to resurrect unfinished issues. I hope you can resolve them in some forum, but at this time I need to be able to have you help me in getting this information or making these decisions.

If angry emotions persist, a physician can ask a family member to leave until he or she can return in a calm manner. The physician can offer to meet with that person individually at another time if that seems helpful.

Violence in the Family

If a patient is concerned about his or her personal safety, interviewing the threatening family members in the room at the same time as the patient is inadvisable. The threat of violence is something to take seriously. The physician can provide the patient a safe environment to explore his or her options. This is true whether it involves a child fearing abuse from a parent or an adult fearing harm from a partner.

Mental Health Referral

Just as a depressed or anxious patient may need a mental health referral, some families dealing with illness may need to be referred for family therapy. The physician may decide to refer the family to a family-oriented mental health professional when certain concerns emerge. If significant anger or conflict erupts between family members and the physician believes this may interfere with the patient's treatment, a family-oriented mental health referral can be useful. Similarly, if the family mentions that the patient's illness has resulted in significant strains or stresses, the physician can offer a family therapy referral to help members cope. Finally, if the family members seem organized around the illness in a way that appears to solidify battlegrounds that were already in place (e.g., a mother so tied to a child's diabetes and its daily routines that she excludes her alienated husband from all interactions with the child and herself), a family therapy referral can potentially help family members resolve conflicts and gain healthier alliances based less on an individual's illness.

FAMILY-ORIENTED INTERVIEW WITH THE INDIVIDUAL PATIENT

Although many benefits accrue from having the family present in the medical interview, the individual patient is often the only one present in either the office or hospital visit. The absence of other family members does not have to lead to a solely individually oriented approach to the patient. If the physician enters the room and sees only an individual, he or she can maintain a family orientation by remembering that this patient is part of a larger context. Several techniques can reinforce this orientation during the interview. First, the physician can gather a family tree or genogram to understand the family health history, the current family members in the patient's context, the stage of the family's life cycle, relationship patterns and how members are involved in the patient's illness, and current family stresses.[9] In addition to gathering the genogram, the physician can ask a series of family-oriented questions that metaphorically bring the family into the office or hospital visit. The following are examples of questions the physician may ask:

Physician: What do other family members think about how you are doing?

or

What does your mother (father, spouse, daughter) believe caused this problem?

or

Has anyone else in the family had a problem like this? How was it treated?

or

Who else in the family is concerned and involved in your problem?

or

Are there other current or recent stresses in your family that are making it difficult to deal with your health care needs?

or

Who in your family can you rely on for help with your current health care needs?

The responses to these questions could alert the physician to the need for recommending that other family members come in for a medical family interview.

CONCLUSION

Working with families in medical practice can be personally and professionally fulfilling. Gaining the skills to work with families contributes to a physician's clinical comfort and effectiveness. Understanding the three functions of a family interview enhances the physician's ability to work with family members in clinical settings. The first function of establishing rapport or joining with family members is fundamental to family interviewing. Gathering information from multiple family members encourages family involvement in the patient's care and provides important information about family beliefs about the illness. Negotiating a treatment plan with the family and educating family members about the illness can improve patient compliance and family confidence in the health care team. Although learning how to interview more than person presents some challenges, the benefits of hearing the multiple perspectives on the cause and treatment of an illness can be invaluable. The family is always part of the treatment team, whether acknowledged by the physician or not. The active inclusion of family members in the treatment team can be a rewarding clinical experience for every physician, regardless of specialty.

REFERENCES

1. Campbell TL: Family's impact on health: a critical review, *Family Systems Medicine* 4:135–228, 1986.
2. Doherty WA, Campbell TL: *Families and health*, Beverly Hills, Calif, 1998, Sage Press.
3. House JS, Landis KR, Umberson D: Social relationships and health, *Science* 241:540–545, 1988.
4. Campbell TL, Patterson JM: The effectiveness of family interventions in the treatment of physical illness, *J Marital Fam Ther* 21:545–584, 1995.
5. Dracup K, Moser DK, Taylor SE, et al: The psychological consequences of cardiopulmonary resuscitation training for family members of patients at risk for sudden death, *Am J Public Health* 87:1434–1439, 1997.
6. Morisky DE, Levine DM, Green LW, et al: Five-year blood pressure control and mortality following health education for hypertensive patients, *Am J Public Health* 73:153–162, 1983.
7. National Heart, Lung and Blood Institute: Management of patient compliance in the treatment of hypertension, *Hypertension* 4:415–423, 1982.
8. Kushner K, Meyer D, Hansen JP: Patients' attitudes toward physician involvement in family conferences, *J Fam Pract* 28:73–78, 1989.
9. McGoldrick M, Gerson S: *Genograms in family assessment*, New York, 1986, Norton Press.

CHAPTER

21 Troubling Personality Styles and Somatization

Because of their troubling personality styles or interpersonal behaviors, some patients are particularly stressful to interview and difficult to manage. Physicians vary greatly in their response. Some interpersonal behaviors are troubling for some physicians and not troubling at all for others. However, a few characteristically troubling types of interpersonal behavior seem difficult for most physicians. These are most often patients who have "difficult" personality traits[1] or who somatize (i.e., patients who have persistent unexplained physical complaints).

Patients with difficult interpersonal behavior or unexplained physical symptoms have been termed "hateful" because they can arouse intensely negative feelings in their physicians.[2] These patients often become the focus of pejorative labels such as "crock," "troll," "turkey," "gomer," or "dirtball." These labels can help relieve physician stress through humor. Such humor comes at a price, however, because the labeling process is dehumanizing and leads to bad care.[3]

The reasons that such patients elicit intense feelings among physicians are complex. In general, however, physicians label a patient when the patient's behavior provokes feelings of anxiety or anger. Demanding, demeaning, angry, or dependent behaviors are examples of the types that lead to labeling. Patients also are labeled when physicians do not know how to help them.

This chapter reviews some of the common causes of troubling interpersonal behavior and discusses some interviewing strategies that can help physicians manage such behavior more successfully. It is hoped that such strategies can help avoid recourse to pejorative labeling. The discussion of each problem is organized under four headings: (1) general characteristics, (2) inner conflicts and needs, (3) stresses of illness and illness behavior, and (4) interviewing strategies.

After the discussion of troubling personality types, suggestions are presented for working with the patient who somatizes. Although troubling interpersonal behavior and somatization are distinct conceptual entities and problems, they are both addressed in this chapter because they commonly overlap in actual practice. Patients with troubling interpersonal behavior often come to their physicians with unexplained or exaggerated physical complaints. Similarly, patients who somatize typically suffer from one or more of the other troubling interpersonal behaviors described in this chapter.

Understanding the general characteristics of troublesome personality types and somatizing patients will help physicians recognize these problems. Through early recognition, physicians can develop appropriate management strategies before falling back on negative labeling, which itself represents a defeat for good care. An awareness of the inner needs and conflicts of these patients can help physicians empathize with them and feel more sympathetic to their underlying distress. The specific suggestions for interviewing strategies can help physicians manage these patients more successfully, facilitate better doctor-patient rapport, and encourage better patient coping, which also will lead to increased physician satisfaction in the management of difficult patients.

It is important to make the distinction between personality traits (or styles) and personality disorders. Many people possess some aspects of the personality styles described here. In psychiatric nomenclature, however, constellations of traits become formal "disorders" only when the traits lead to persistent maladaptive behavior that compromises functioning.[4] Furthermore, when such patients develop a bona fide acute or chronic general medical illness, the stresses of the general medical illness usually exacerbate their troubling interpersonal behaviors or tendencies to somatize.

COMPULSIVE PATIENTS

General Characteristics

Compulsive individuals tend to be concerned about details and lead rigid, highly structured, and predictable lives. Such people emphasize rational processes and disdain emotionality. They often pride themselves on their ability to solve problems. They like to break problems into manageable segments and solve them methodically, one by one. In the words of Sergeant Friday, compulsive individuals may ask for "the facts, and only the facts."

Compulsive individuals function best when they feel in control of themselves and their circumstances or the people around them. In lieu of control, these individuals strive for certainty. They avoid ambiguity at all costs.

Inner Conflicts and Needs

Compulsive people feel threatened or anxious when confronted by ambiguity, uncertainty, or emotionality. They often experience inner conflict around the recognition and expression of their own emotional lives. Feelings of anger, anxiety, or sadness are often denied, displaced, projected onto others, or experienced as physical sensations such as pain (somatization). These processes often occur unconsciously. The compulsive person may honestly insist that he or she feels no anger, when it is obvious to others that anger is present.

It is probably this fear of their own inner emotional lives that leads compulsive individuals to favor rationality and control. The compulsive individual desires control of self, others, and events. When adequate levels of control are ensured, the compulsive person feels more secure and enjoys an increased sense of well-being.

Stresses of Illness and Illness Behavior

Illness creates special anxiety for the compulsive individual. The uncertainty of illness strikes at the core of the individual's strategy for life adjustment. This person can no longer count on rationality to solve life's problems. No longer can he or she predict what will happen day by day. The emotions associated with illness—anxiety, sadness, and anger—are themselves anathema to the compulsive patient.

The anxiety a compulsive patient experiences during illness may lead to a doubly difficult situation. The physical symptoms of illness are frightening to anyone because they present uncertainty. However, the compulsive patient is independently frightened by the emergence of disquieting symptoms because they represent loss of control. The loss of control itself engenders high anxiety. Such a state of high arousal amplifies the illness symptoms and brings physical symptoms of its own, creating a cycle that may be difficult to break.

Under the stress of illness the compulsive patient develops an embattled stance to attain—or rather regain—control. In the battle for control the patient may see not only the disease but also the people involved in his or her care as potential enemies. This can lead to many conflicts with the physician, the nurses, family, and friends, often over seemingly insignificant issues.

The compulsive patient needs and desires information. If the information provided does not resolve enough of the uncertainty, the demand for more information can become insatiable. Question asking becomes repetitive and circular in a desperate attempt to gain control. Submitting to a hospital routine can be humiliating for compulsive patients, and they often fight for control of minor and seemingly irrelevant details, such as insisting that a sleeping pill be delivered at 9:30 instead of 10:00.

Interviewing Strategies

Compulsive patients, even more than other patients, must be treated as equal partners in the alliance against illness. Detailed, accurate, and specific information is essential for good coping by compulsive individuals. This information should be provided in as straightforward a manner as possible. The physician must be scrupulously honest, but care should be taken not to overemphasize the uncertainties of treatments or responses.

The physician should allow the patient as much control as possible in the planning of every stage of treatment. The options and recommendations should be presented, and the patient should be allowed to make as many choices as possible. When compulsive patients are hospitalized, every reasonable effort should be made to minimize the enforced dependency that accompanies patient status.

Compulsive patients must not be prematurely reassured. Unrealistic reassurance that is not based on accurate factual investigations will create more anxiety and mistrust. In general, such patients will not react well to a "fatherly" arm around the shoulder, a pat on the head, or the global, "Do not worry, everything will turn out OK."

Compulsive personality traits can interfere with patient management because patients are so frightened by uncertainty that they continue to ask repetitive questions, do not seem to listen to the answers, and become angry when providers get frustrated and begin to cut their answers short. Sometimes this drives compulsive patients to accuse doctors of "not listening" or "not caring" or "not explaining." In reality the physician may have spent a great deal of time and effort attempting to discuss the illness with the patient. However, when the answers never seemed sufficient, the physician may have become irritated and said such things as, "I just told you the answer to that question. You're not listening."

This type of physician comment usually raises the patient's anxiety and creates dissonance in the relationship. A far better type of physician response addresses the patient's underlying anxiety about the uncertainty of the illness situation. For example, faced with interminable questions, a physician might say something such as the following:

> **Physician:** No matter how much information I give you, I don't seem to be able to provide you with what you're really looking for. Is there some other question that you might want to ask but that you haven't been able to ask yet?

Or a physician might say something like this:

> **Physician:** I don't seem to be able to provide you with as much information as you need. I have a feeling that this whole situation is simply very troubling for you, especially the uncertainty. You appear to be a type of person who likes to be able to understand what is happening and to know where things are heading. Being sick, with all its uncertainties, is very difficult.

When the physician addresses the patient's underlying anxiety in this way, the patient may be able to begin talking about underlying fears and recognize that the uncertainty and lack of control may be particularly disabling. Simply recognizing the source of this distress can be a relief in many instances and can actually help the patient cope.

DEPENDENT PATIENTS

General Characteristics

As implied by the label, the dependent person finds life difficult to negotiate without outside assistance. Other people, usually one or more "special" people, are sought out to provide a steady fount of emotional support, as well as to help manage day-to-day affairs and important decisions. When this help and support is not delivered, the dependent person may feel deserted, hurt, and angry and may demand more assistance.

Inner Conflicts and Needs

The dependent person has powerful needs to be nurtured and protected because of underlying fears of rejection and of being alone. The active caring and help of others provide comfort and relief from insecurity, but only temporarily. Thus the dependent patient's search for support can be relentless. As these demands for support escalate, the dependent person can, in a self-defeating manner, evoke the very rejection that was most feared in the first place.

Stresses of Illness and Illness Behavior

Illness is specially frightening for dependent people because they not only suffer the normal worries that illness brings but also imagine that sickness will lead to a loss of love. This added anxiety can lead to increased and exaggerated dependency on their usual caretakers and to increased physical symptoms (somatization).

Dependent individuals often turn to their physicians and other health care providers to fulfill their general dependency needs, as well as to relieve the specific anxieties evoked by illness. Providers often accept and welcome this dependency at first, especially if (as is often the case) the dependent person expresses a great deal of gratitude. Dependent patients often thank their physicians profusely and make comments like this one:

Patient: Thank you so much for listening. You're the only doctor I've ever had who really understands.

Some physicians feel proud to evoke such praise from their patients, but experienced caregivers learn that such laudatory testimonials often lead to later disappointments. Once such patients have become emotionally dependent on their doctors, they tend to experience persistent physical symptoms because of their fear of losing access to the doctor's care and attention. This process is often unconscious (true somatization) or only partly conscious. The nature and severity of the symptoms will become increasingly difficult to explain in purely physical terms. Thus the brief honeymoon between the satisfied patient and the doctor will come to an end as the doctor becomes increasingly puzzled and then frustrated and exasperated. Sensing this, the patient will become yet more afraid of losing the nurturing relationship and will often become even more clinging and demanding, which only makes matters worse. In this way, such patients may change from a physician's dream to a physician's nightmare.

Interviewing Strategies

The dependent patient certainly needs to be nurtured. Any attempt to treat the dependent patient as an independent partner in the doctor-patient relationship will usually fail and lead the patient to feel rejected and to try to find another doctor who will really "care." Thus a "parental" stance of reassurance can often be successful with dependent patients.

When dependent patients become demanding or clingy, physicians must make special efforts to limit the patients' demands in a gentle and supportive way that minimizes the patient's inference of rejection. Physicians should state their concern and caring very explicitly at the time that limits also are set clearly. For example:

> **Physician:** I want you to know that I am concerned about your health, and I want to do everything I can to get you better and also to help support you through this difficult period. But I also need to let you know that I won't be able to spend forty-five minutes with you every time we get together. I understand that this time has been helpful to you, but I can't spend this amount of time with you and also get everything else done that I need to do. I would like to spend about fifteen minutes with you each time you come for a check-up. How does that sound to you?

Because dependent patients will almost always interpret any firm limits as a rejection, it may be helpful for the physician to warn the patient to anticipate this feeling. The physician might say something like this:

> **Physician:** It occurs to me that trying to keep to 15 minutes might make you feel bad, perhaps a little rejected. I am sorry if you feel this way, because I am not rejecting you. I'm just trying to let

you know the framework around which I think I can be of most help.

Scheduling periodic visits that are independent of physical symptoms is another helpful strategy. This gives the patient the assurance of having at least some ongoing support without needing to be ill.

Physician: To give you more effective support, I would like to see you regularly for a while, regardless of whether your symptoms are better or worse. I suggest once a week to start with. What do you think?

The frequency of such visits may need to be quite high initially to break the circle of symptoms to anxiety to dependency to symptoms. Once this circle is broken, the frequency of visits can usually be progressively lowered, and often the visits can be phased out altogether.

Regardless of attempts by the physician to engage the patient in a healthy dialogue about the dependency, the extremely dependent patient will continue to test the limits of the physician's support. Even if the intervention described above seems to be helpful in the beginning, some dependent patients feel insatiable neediness and will continue to ask for more than can be reasonably given. The challenge for the physician is to continue to set appropriate limits without becoming so angry or rejecting that the patient is frightened or forced away.

HISTRIONIC PATIENTS

General Characteristics

Histrionic patients, also called "hysterical" patients, live life at a high emotional pitch. Most experiences, including illness, are intense for them, and they can vacillate rapidly between emotional and giddy "highs" and very distressed "lows." They are often attractive and seductive in the emotional, interpersonal, and sexual sense. They can be flashy in the way they behave, as well as the way they dress, walk, and talk. Their emotionality is usually labile and is often perceived by others as shallow.

Inner Conflicts and Needs

Histrionic individuals are driven by a need for admiration as a substitute for love. They tend to confuse admiration with love, which they may not be able to recognize in any other form. At a deeper, usually unconscious, level they crave love and fear that they are unlovable. Histrionic women in male company will often flaunt their sexuality in their efforts to receive admiration from men in lieu of more meaningful intimacy.

Histrionic men, depending on the circumstances, may use flirtation or displays of bravado, humor, or aggressiveness in their efforts to seek admiration.

Stresses of Illness and Illness Behavior

Even mild illness is likely to be an intense experience for histrionic patients. In addition to the concerns that any sick person is likely to feel, histrionic patients may feel a special threat to their physical attractiveness, on which they depend for their attention. When histrionic individuals become sick, they therefore make special efforts to gain the attention, caring, and affection of caregivers. These efforts may include exaggerated and dramatic accounts of their illness, grandiose and inappropriate compliments to the physician, attempts to present themselves only in the best light, and, if the physician is of the opposite sex, seductive dress and behavior. Male histrionic patients may attempt to intimidate the physician, especially if the physician is also male. The description of their symptoms will often be dramatic and intense. This is partly because they experience the symptoms intensely, but also because of their need for maximum admiration and sympathy from the physician. This amplification of symptoms may be partly or even entirely unconscious (somatization).

Interviewing Strategies

The physician can help histrionic patients cope by appropriately admiring them when they demonstrate this need. Care must be taken to avoid any behavior that might be interpreted by patients as seductive, challenging, or belittling. If patients make sexual overtures, these must be politely refused. For example:

> **Physician:** Thank you for your interest in me. I am flattered, but I need to keep our relationship a professional one. I think I can be of most help to you that way. I hope that is OK with you.

If the patient makes threats or in other ways tries to be intimidating in pursuing his or her demands, the best policy is usually for the physician to show respect and seek further exploration before considering a definitive response. In this way the physician can often avoid either confronting or conceding to a threat. For example:

> **Physician:** I can see you feel very strongly about this, and I respect that. Tell me more about what makes this such an important issue for you. If I can fully understand your needs and wishes, I expect we can find a way to help.

The excessive somatic complaints of the histrionic patient may be reduced if the physician shows specific respect for, and interest in, the ways in which the patient copes with the discomfort he or she experiences:

Physician: I want you to know that I think you're doing a good job coping, given the pain you're experiencing. (Respect)
We'll do all we can to figure this out and get you better as soon as possible. (Support)
Tell me more about the ways in which you've managed to keep going in spite of all these troubles.

SELF-DEFEATING (MASOCHISTIC) PATIENTS

General Characteristics

Self-defeating, or masochistic, patients suffer in life and need to continue to experience this suffering. They perceive themselves as always giving to others and always suffering. This need to suffer, however, is not the same as a need to be physically hurt. Self-defeating patients may become "addicted" to a career of self-sacrifice and suffering, but they do not actually seek pain, physical abuse, or punishment.

Inner Conflicts and Needs

Masochistic patients have a psychological need to maintain the role of sufferer. Perhaps because of unconscious guilt or identification with long-suffering parents,[5] self-defeating patients are not able to escape from their suffering. They have a strong need to see themselves as self-sacrificing and suffering because otherwise they would have to face intolerable emotions such as hatred of a loved one or guilt or failure. The prospect of recovery or relief from suffering presents a conflict to such patients. Recovery is tempting because the suffering is real, but it is frightening because it would bring painful emotions and drastic changes of lifestyle.

Stresses of Illness and Illness Behavior

Long-suffering individuals adapt well to illness but may be threatened by recovery. They can adapt well to the sick role behavior but not so well to recovery. Such patients readily adopt sick role behaviors even when they have only mild physical illnesses or none at all.

Masochistic patients often frustrate physicians because the patients do not seem to desire to get well. Whatever the doctor attempts does not seem to work. Such patients have been called "manipulative help rejecters" because nothing a physician can do ever seems to help.[2]

Interviewing Strategies

When working with self-defeating personalities in the medical setting, it is important for the physician to respect their suffering and to be wary of promising a complete cure. The physician should remember that illness is a way of life and that the threat of an illness-free life is unconsciously troubling for these patients. Such patients genuinely suffer and do not consciously thwart attempts at recovery. Their symptoms may be caused mostly by somatization but are nevertheless real. Patients in this condition really do feel terrible and are unaware of their need to remain ill.

In general, a useful intervention strategy includes a physician's explanation that medical science has not been able to find a complete answer to all problems for all patients. The emphasis for the future should probably be away from any notion of complete "cure" and toward the notion of "coping." Medications or other therapies might help to some degree, but the cornerstone of effective treatment should become the scheduling of regular appointments to check on general conditions and to focus on the patient's ability to function despite the physical problems. As always, the physician must keep an open mind and watch for any new physical signs that warrant further investigation.

The physician should never promise cures or complete relief from suffering because such hopes will usually be dashed and lead to frustration for the patient and for the physician. In addition, patients should not be told to, "Come back again when you feel sick," because this invites the patient to again use illness behavior to get attention from the physician. The patient should be encouraged to return to regularly scheduled appointments, "whether or not you feel sick." This strategy has been shown to decrease overall medical costs and hospital use for many patients with multiple, chronic, unexplained somatic complaints.[6]

This conservative management approach will not always lead to an easy doctor-patient relationship. Many self-defeating patients continue to suffer and have physical crises again and again. However, a physician who can set appropriate limits in a supportive way and stay with the patient for the long haul will be able to limit iatrogenic injuries, decrease medical care abuse, and contribute to the overall adaptation of long-suffering patients.

BORDERLINE PATIENTS

General Characteristics

The term *borderline* refers to a group of patients with a relatively persistent set of personality characteristics, the hallmarks of which are instability in personal relationships, unstable moods, and impulsive behavior. This is a seriously disabling personality disorder. While the name historically described a syndrome of psychopathology at the border of severity between neurosis and psychosis, the concept is now used to describe a group of patients who simply demonstrate the characteristics described above in a marked and persistent way.

The patient with borderline pathology commonly experiences wide fluctuations of feeling in intimate relationships—intense affection and love alternating with disgust or hatred. This seesaw quality in the borderline patient's close relationships carries itself to other situations and to other relationships, including the relationship with the physician. The alternating feelings of love and hatred toward others mirror feelings the borderline patient has toward himself or herself.

In addition to the characteristic vacillation of feelings toward self and others, borderline patients suffer from extreme mood swings, an inability to tolerate being alone, difficulty in completing tasks, and impulsive behavior. While many patients possess some of these features, borderline patients demonstrate these problems to such a degree and with such intensity that a separate label is appropriate to help understand them and to develop appropriate intervention strategies.

Inner Conflicts and Needs

Borderline patients feel unloved and threatened by people and circumstances. These feelings may derive from early psychic trauma, including insufficient emotional support from parental figures,[7] or from a lack of resolution of very early or traumatic childhood conflicts (i.e., before the age of 18 months).[8] Borderline patients need emotional support and consistency in their relationships with others, but their internal psychic distress and fluctuating temperament lead to characteristic interpersonal failures. As with the dependent personality, the interpersonal demands of the borderline patient often lead to the very rejection so feared in the beginning. This rejection then proves to such patients that the world is unreliable and unloving. This tragic circle of neediness, rejection, and bitterness in close interpersonal relationships can be recreated in the doctor-patient or staff-patient relationship when the borderline patient becomes sick.[9]

Stresses of Illness and Illness Behavior

Illness presents special adaptive challenges to the borderline patient. In a world that is perceived as unreliable and threatening, illness or hospitalization becomes a stress that threatens further loss of love and support. The ability to tolerate anxiety, frustration, pain, or uncertainty may be severely challenged in the borderline patient with limited resources to cope. The tendency to vacillate between good and bad extremes can become intensified. The fear of being alone becomes more severe, and the tendency toward impulsive behavior can grow excessively.

The borderline patient may describe the physician or other staff in glowing terms one day and hate them the next. These dramatic variations may occur in response to trivial incidents of which the staff and the physician are unaware. Equally dramatic changes may occur in the severity of the patient's symptomatic complaints, since these are greatly affected by whether the patient feels loved or hated at the time. These changes in symptoms, at least partly caused by somatization of negative emotions, may be difficult to explain on purely physical grounds and therefore will puzzle the physician. Furthermore, the borderline patient usually has little insight into his or her own exquisite sensitivity; borderline patients characteristically hold others primarily responsible for their own emotional state and often for their symptoms as well.

Interviewing Strategies

Depending on the severity of the borderline pathology, the ability to develop therapeutic doctor-patient relationships can vary greatly. Nevertheless, the following general guidelines can be helpful.

Perhaps the most useful principle is to remember that borderline patients are like frightened children. They have a fear of the unknown, of strangers, and of illness that is akin to a child's fearfulness but that may be masked by more adult presentations of anger, demandingness, and bitterness. Attempts to understand the "frightened child" behind the storm of emotionality will help the physician manage his or her own feelings and develop a strategy for helping patients. The best strategy, just as with children, is to combine consistent support with firm structure and limit setting.

The borderline patient feels a deep and continuing need for reassurance. Thus supportive attention and concern can be soothing, although the emotional "supplies" that the physician possesses may be insufficient for the patient's needs. When these needs and demands escalate, the physician should try to be as supportive as possible but to maintain a firm sense of the limits of his or her own tolerance, as well as the limits of the hospital environment. If the demands are presented with threats or aggressiveness, the best response is usually along the lines already described for histrionic patients. The patient's legitimate concerns and fears should be addressed, but when unreasonable demands are made, the physician should set limits in as clear and supportive a way as possible. At times there may be no way to completely satisfy a borderline patient (just as there may be no way to meet all the requests of a demanding child). However, sensitive attention to the patient's underlying fear and insecurity may communicate enough support to facilitate more adaptive behavior on the patient's part.

Some other strategies may be helpful in the management of the borderline patient, especially in the hospital environment. Since the borderline patient is often frightened of being alone, it can be helpful for his or her room to be positioned near the nursing station and for nurses or other staff to make frequent room checks. It has also proved useful for one staff member to be assigned the task of communicating medical information to the patient and for discussing problems. Because the borderline patient can "split" medical providers into ones they see as "good" and others who are "bad," limiting medical and problem discussion to one provider can minimize the tendency for distortion in communication to occur and can also minimize the danger of intense emotional reactions to different caregivers or from different providers.[9] Specially called staff meetings may be helpful to develop a unified care plan for particularly disruptive borderline patients.

NARCISSISTIC PATIENTS

General Characteristics

Patients with narcissistic personality traits feel that they have special qualities and experiences and are entitled to special attention and special treatment.[4] This is their perspective about illness, just as it is about all other aspects of life. They seem genuinely perplexed when their sense of entitlement is challenged. It is as if their expectation for special treatment is their birthright and they expect others to recognize this right implicitly, in the same way that they recognize it for themselves. Some patients with narcissistic features are from the upper socioeconomic class or are leaders in business, politics, religion, or the military. Their expectations for special treatment may thus be based on realistic experiences. However, most narcissistic individuals develop and retain their sense of entitlement even when the world has not acknowledged their uniqueness.

Narcissistic individuals generally cannot understand others' points of view. They can be so wrapped up in their own world of uniqueness and expectation that every experience is filtered and colored by their own point of view. They have little tolerance or flexibility for the reality of the functioning of complex social systems. They expect rules, policies, or procedures to be waived for their personal desires or comforts, and they become enraged at the thought of being treated like everyone else.

Inner Conflicts and Needs

Narcissistic personality traits and, especially, narcissistic personality disorders generally are built on an edifice of insecurity and ego deficits. Narcissists' self-esteem is actually extremely fragile, and their apparent self-confidence depends on the adoration, respect, or uniqueness with which others treat them. The overarching need is to be respected and treated as special.

Inner conflicts revolve around this insecurity about self-worth. These conflicts may be well defended, and narcissists are often unaware of their fragile self-esteem. This shaky self-esteem may become apparent to patients only when they are threatened by the loss of special treatment by the social world. When respect and uniqueness is lost or denied, narcissists may react with rage or depression.

Stresses of Illness and Illness Behavior

Illness and hospitalization present great threats to narcissists because illness confronts these patients with their own vulnerability. Narcissistic patients who become sick participate in a living nightmare; they feel powerless and lost in a system that cannot be controlled and that often treats them in the manner they most fear, as one of many. This can arouse primitive, childlike fears of abandonment and, in general, a loss of love. Narcissists' usual sense of self-confidence and pride can be deeply shaken. These patients may be tempted to elaborate or exaggerate their symptoms in order to establish their unique status. This may happen unconsciously (somatization) or consciously (factitious illness).

As narcissistic defenses become challenged, patients may react with depression and with rage at a medical system that refuses to treat them as special. Narcissists may also feel this rage against particular providers or institutions if they feel that the uniqueness of their symptoms and entitlement has not been recognized. This rage can present in the form of impractical or impossible demands on the system or in the form of bitter criticism about alleged failures of diagnosis or treatment. Narcissists may also be depressed about the threatened loss of esteem, efficacy, and power in the world.

Interviewing Strategies

The treatment of the narcissistic patient presents a great challenge to the physician and to the health care system in general. When this patient is articulate, educated, and powerful, the rage and implied threat (sometimes of lawsuits) can frighten the caregiver. The physicians and other caregivers may change their general procedures in ways that may compromise good care. On the other hand, some caregivers may never "give anything" to the narcissistic patient, because some physicians may not want to be "manipulated" and do not want to cede one iota of control to the patient, especially to an unreasonably demanding one.

An intermediate strategy between the two extremes may be helpful. First of all, the physician should understand the underlying fear of the narcissistic patient. This fear is greater than that of the average patient. Not only is the narcissistic patient afraid of all the normal events that might occur in illness, but the narcissistic patient suffers additional fear because of the loss of uniqueness that illness implies. When a hospital environment treats a patient as "one among many," the narcissist suffers a special humiliation that must be understood before he or she can be helped.

The general strategy suggested in this text focuses on supporting the patient's claim to uniqueness, within the limits that the system and physician can tolerate. It is usually helpful to ask the angry, demanding patient what specific changes would make him or her happier. If the requests are general, such as, "I just want to be treated with more respect," an attempt should be made to get the patient to be quite specific in these requests. Once a series of requests has been received, the physician or staff can try to meet as many of these requests as possible. This often temporarily mollifies the narcissistic patient. Some but not all of the requests can usually be reasonably met. The patient can be told this directly. For example:

Physician: We can change the time that the blood pressures are taken in the night so you can get a better night's sleep. I will write a specific, special order to make sure that this occurs. I can also make sure that the visiting hours for your son are changed so that he can come visit you when he gets out of work. I won't be able to change the meal times, however, because the dietary service is obligated to deliver to this ward according to a fixed schedule.

Furthermore, if the physician can meet some of these requests, he or she can often negotiate for some relaxation of the patient's difficult behaviors. For example:

Physician: I have discussed your requests with the nurses. As I mentioned, there are several requests that we can happily meet, but a few that just can't work out. In return for our efforts to meet your special needs, I wonder if you would be willing save your requests and problems for discussion with the head nurse, who will come to see you every day between 1 and 2 PM. If you discuss these requests with every staff member who comes in, the hospital routine can get confused and disrupted.

SOMATIZATION

General Characteristics

Somatization has been defined as "the expression of emotional discomfort and psychosocial distress in the language of bodily symptoms."[10] By this definition, "emotional discomfort" includes emotional distress, as well as bona fide mental syndromes or disorders such as major depression or panic disorder. In most cases of somatization, the sufferer is entirely unaware of the psychologic or neurobiologic connection between the emotional psychiatric dysfunction and the experience of physical illness.[11]

It is of utmost importance that physicians understand that the physical suffering of somatizing patients is just as real as suffering that has a demonstrable pathophysiologic etiology. Furthermore, from a differential diagnostic or management point of view, *the patient's response to placebo is of no use in determining whether pain complaints are psychogenic or physical in etiology.* Some physical pain responds to placebo, and some psychogenic pain does not. For example, 30% of postoperative surgical pain responds to placebo.[12] Thus physicians should not conceptualize the somatization process (or psychogenic pain) as "all in the head" or "not real." This trivializes serious problems and implies conscious deception in a situation in which the patient's experience of the pain is real.

The physician should distinguish between somatization (which is an *unconscious* process, of which the patient is unaware) and certain other related syndromes in which physical symptoms are *consciously* manufactured. "Malingering" refers to the process of consciously producing or exaggerating physical symptoms in the effort to achieve some understandable external gain—for example, disability benefits, insurance claims, or potent analgesics. The rare and often very dramatic and self-destructive Munchhausen's syndrome (also known as factitious disorder) involves the conscious production of symptoms in response to a compelling psychologic drive to be a patient.

Inner Conflicts and Needs

In contrast to many of the troubling interpersonal behaviors described previously, somatization represents a final common pathway for numerous different forms of psychic disturbance. Some mental disorders, such as depression or panic disorder, are associated with demonstrable neurobiologic substrates.[13] In such conditions, the mind-body connection may lead to direct physical manifestations of the psychiatric problem, such as insomnia and fatigue. Such symptoms usually respond well to appropriate psychotropic medication (or, sometimes, targeted psychotherapy). For other somatizing patients, complex psychologic mechanisms play a psychodynamic or behaviorally conditioned role in perpetuating physical symptoms and interpersonal dysfunction.

In all cases somatizing patients experience genuine and distressing physical symptoms, of which the cause is obscure. As a rule, somatizing patients are eager to find explanations for their suffering and consume considerable amounts of medical time and resources in seeking answers. Such patients often remain dissatisfied with their care. Because of the intractable and persistent nature of their physical symptoms and their demands for relief, physicians often find them troubling to manage.[1]

Somatizing patients are stuck in a painful trap; they need and want relief, but they characteristically find it difficult to accept explanations or treatments of their symptoms that are based on an appropriate psychobiologic understanding of mind-body relationships.

Successful management of the somatizing patient usually requires that the physician possess considerable knowledge and skill. Besides mastering the knowledge base for appropriate assessment, the physician who attempts treatment of the somatizing patient must develop a highly effective set of communication skills for rapport development and partnership for treatment.

Stresses of Illness and Illness Behavior

Patients who somatize may also develop concomitant physical illnesses. Management of the somatizing patient usually becomes more difficult in the face of clear-cut physical illness. The tendency to somatize may persist, resulting in the amplification of symptoms that have been caused by an underlying physical illness.[14] This creates circular problems and increasing confusion and frustration for both the patient and the doctor.

In the context of an emergent and definable pathologic condition, there is often increasing pressure for both the patient and the doctor to latch onto any positive physical finding, however obscure, in the hope that it will provide a complete explanation for the symptoms. By the same token, there is the related pressure to try any physical treatment that seems even marginally relevant in the hope that it will provide a cure. Because of these pressures, physicians often undertake risky investigations and treatments of marginal relevance. Such investigations and treatments often lead to iatrogenic damage, both psychologic and physical.

Interviewing Strategies

Many doctors find it difficult to deal with somatization. Even when physicians believe that somatization may be the principal problem, many find themselves colluding with somatizing patients in an endless series of physical investigations and specialist opinions. This fruitless search for answers has the effect of reinforcing patients' determination to find purely physical explanations. By the time the physician decides to call a halt to this process, it is virtually impossible to do so without alienating the patient.

Despite having the "benefit" of frequent unsatisfactory clinical experiences, such as that described in the preceding paragraph, most physicians feel unable to develop management strategies that can lead to better outcomes. On the other hand, physicians who recognize the possibility or probability of somatization early in the assessment process can implement an appropriate management strategy before iatrogenic damage has been done and before the physician-patient relationship has deteriorated beyond repair.

A communication and intervention strategy that incorporates the five steps described below can be readily learned and effectively used by non-psychiatrists.[15]

1. *Diagnose and treat depression and anxiety* when they are present. Up to 50% of patients with severe somatization have comorbid depression or anxiety disorders. As described in Chapter 16, management of somatization becomes less complex when these psychiatric syndromes are effectively treated (with medications or psychotherapy).
2. *Develop rapport.* Understand and empathize with the patient and his or her dilemma.
3. *Change the agenda.* Emphasize *coping,* not *curing.*
4. *See the patient regularly,* whether or not he or she is experiencing the physical problems.
5. *"Don't just do something, stand there!"*[16]

Developing Rapport

Developing rapport requires physicians to try their best to experience the world from the point of view of the somatizing—but suffering—patient. Physicians must acquire a vivid and accurate picture of the symptoms themselves but do so while moving quickly toward understanding (and empathizing with) the effect of these symptoms on the patient's overall quality of life.

When interviewing somatizing patients, it is always important to start with the symptoms themselves, but also to make it clear from an early stage that the physician is interested in the impact of these symptoms on the patient's life.

> **Physician:** I would like to hear more detail about your symptoms, starting with the first thing that went wrong and what the circumstances were when it happened.

After listening to the patient's story, it is essential to empathize with the patient's suffering. The physician can do this by recognizing the patient's distress and legitimizing his or her suffering. This is important to developing an effective partnership with the patient.

When developing an effective partnership, the physician should never say, or even imply, that "there is nothing wrong" or that "it's all in the mind." Somatizing patients know there is something wrong, and they derive little comfort from being told that there is nothing wrong. This discounts their suffering and serves as a marker for lack of physician understanding. Physicians can and should make comments such as the following:

> **Physician:** It is clear to me that these are very uncomfortable symptoms. (reflection)
> I can well understand how distressed you have been about them. (legitimation)

Somatizing patients are typically frustrated by the medical care system, which has not produced any relief from suffering. Empathizing with this frustration can serve as an important building block for the relationship. For example:

> **Physician:** I can certainly understand why you are so frustrated with doctors. You've been suffering with the stomach trouble for five years, and yet you cannot find anyone who has been able to tell you what is wrong and what you can do for relief. (legitimation)

Part of the empathic process involves understanding the somatizing patient's life situation and fears regarding causation. When beginning the assessment of psychosocial issues with a somatizing patient, it is always best to first ask about the *effects* of the symptoms on the patient's emotional state and day-to-day activities. Without this introduction, somatizing patients may feel that the physician is discounting the physical suffering if the focus is turned onto the psychosocial life situation. The following approach often proves useful:

> **Physician:** These are tough symptoms. How have they affected your day-to-day life (e.g., work, home life, relationships, sleep, energy, sex life, or mood)?

Similarly, accurate empathy requires understanding the nature of the patient's concerns about etiology:

> **Physician:** It would help me if you could let me know about your own thoughts and fears about the possible causes of these symptoms.

When physicians elicit a patient's underlying concerns, it is essential to empathize with these concerns and, when possible, to offer clear, realistic reassurance:

> **Physician:** I can well understand why you might suspect that and how worrying that would be. (legitimation)

> Based on the history, the physical examinations, and the other studies we have done, I can tell you emphatically (and our consultants agree) that your symptoms are not due to underlying heart disease (or cancer).
> Let me review, again, my specific reasons for saying this. (reassurance)

Changing the Agenda

Changing the agenda requires introducing a change in the mindset of both the patient and the physician to focus on coping, not curing. This requires accepting that the symptoms are of a chronic nature and are essentially not life threatening. Acute interventions have not worked in the past, so the management of symptoms through coping mechanisms is the best strategy.

Seeing the Patient Regularly

Physicians must schedule regular visits with patients to monitor symptoms, to assess the effect of symptoms on the patients' quality of life, and to develop the interpersonal relationships that will help patients cope better with their chronic symptoms. Since somatizing patients often develop their symptoms under circumstances of high stress and since they tend to use physicians as a significant source of social support, an alteration in this maladaptive cycle can be extremely effective. The physician should not wait for patients to develop new symptoms. Patients with chronic, unexplained symptoms need to be seen regularly, usually about once a month, whether or not they are experiencing their symptoms. When physicians are able to maintain a relationship with these patients and see them regularly, the psychosocial aspects of the patients' conditions often become more apparent. The intensity and severity of their physical problems often diminish.

"Don't Just Do Something, Stand There!"

It is important for the physician to minimize new investigations; however, somatizing patients will often demand new tests. Sometimes it will be appropriate to agree to more tests, but more often it will be better to say something that both deflects the patient from further investigation, at least for the time being, and gently introduces the possibility of a different approach. This is perhaps the most delicate and complex intervention of the whole process. Although this intervention naturally has to be tailored to each patient, it might be something like the following interchange between the physician and the patient:

Physician: I can well understand your wish for further tests because naturally you hope that they might provide a definite explanation for your symptoms and therefore some hope of relief. Sadly, I have to tell you that the chance of further tests showing even a partial explanation is virtually zero. I feel confident of this, and all the consultants you have seen agree.

Patient: So what do you suggest? I know something is the matter.

Physician: What I suggest is that we agree to have a temporary halt to the tests while we review the situation, watch you very closely, and consider a different approach that I think can offer at least a partial solution. At the moment, I feel that all the information we have from our tests and our consultants make it clear that we are not dealing with a dangerous medical condition that we are missing. Since I understand how much you are suffering and how these problems are affecting your daily life, I would like to see you regularly to help work out a way to manage these symptoms better. I will offer suggestions for treatment strategies that might be helpful, but I think we both have to understand that the goal right now is not one of complete cure. Rather, we are shooting for some slight improvements and for ways to help you cope better with the problem. The most important part is that I would like to see you regularly to monitor your progress and work with you to help with treatment approaches.

This type of conservative management of chronic, unexplained physical complaints, using the doctor-patient relationship as the key ingredient for "treatment," has been shown in randomized, prospective clinical trials to be effective in achieving improved clinical outcome and decreased medical expenditures.[17]

CONCLUSION

Numerous clinical situations involve troubling interpersonal behavior or chronic somatization that has the potential to cause great distress for physicians and poor clinical results for patients. Interviewing strategies based on understanding the determinants of these troubling behaviors and somatization can be effective for patient management and rewarding for the patient and the physician alike.

REFERENCES

1. Hahn S, Kroenke K, Spitzer RL, et al: The difficult patient: prevalence, psychopathology, and functional impairment, *J Gen Intern Med* 11(1):1–8, 1996.
2. Groves JE: Taking care of the hateful patient, *N Engl J Med*, 298(16):883–887, 1978.

3. Cohen-Cole SA, Friedman CP: The language problem: integration of psychosocial variables into routine medical care, *Psychosomatics* 24:54, 1983.
4. American Psychiatric Association: *Diagnostic and statistical manual of mental disorders*, ed 4, Washington, DC, 1994, The Association.
5. Levy ST, Lyle C, Cohen-Cole SA: Masochistic character pathology in medical settings. In Ross JM, Myers WA, editors: *Psychoanalytic psychotherapy*, Washington, DC, 1988, American Psychiatric Association.
6. Smith GR, Monson RA, Ray DC: Psychiatric consultation in somatization disorder: a randomized controlled study, *N Engl J Med* 314:1407–1413, 1986.
7. Adler G: *Borderline psychopathology and its treatment*, New York, 1985, Jason Aronson.
8. Kernberg O: *Object relations theory and clinical psychoanalysis*, New York, 1976, Jason Aronson.
9. Groves JE: Management of the borderline patient on a medical-surgical ward: the psychiatric consultant's role, *Int J Psychiatry Med* 6:337–348, 1975.
10. Katon W, Ries RK, Kleinman A: The prevalence of somatization in primary care, *Comp Psychiatry* 25:208–215, 1984.
11. Walker EA, Unetzer J, Katon WJ: Understanding and caring for the distressed patient with multiple unexplained symptoms, *J Am Board Fam Pract* 11(5):347–356, 1998.
12. Ford CV: *The somatizing disorders: illness as a way of life*, New York, 1983, Elsevier Science Publishing.
13. Cole: Depression. In Noble J, editor: *Primary care medicine*, ed 3 Mosby, in press.
14. Barsky AJ: Amplification, somatization, and the somatoform disorders, *Psychosomatics* 33(1):28–34, 1992.
15. Gask L, Goldberg D, Porter R, et al: The treatment of somatization: the evaluation of a training package with general practice trainees, *J Psychosom Res* 33:697–703, 1989.
16. Drossman: The problem patient: evaluation and care of medical patients with psychosocial disturbances, *Ann Intern Med* 88(3):366–372, 1978.
17. Smith GR, Monson RA, Ray DC: Psychiatric consultation in somatization disorder: a randomized controlled study, *N Engl J Med* 314:1407–1413, 1986.

CHAPTER

22 Nonadherence, Lifestyle Change, Stress, and Support

Chapter 21 reviews communication difficulties that arise when the physician deals with problems of personality, which also are often associated with unexplained physical symptoms. This chapter discusses communication difficulties concerning problems of nonadherence, lifestyle, stress, and support. The chapter starts with a general overview of nonadherence and then discusses medication nonadherence in particular. Following the discussion of medication nonadherence, the chapter considers six lifestyle situations that carry health risks and are often associated with nonadherence. The first four are negative health habits: alcohol and substance abuse, smoking, obesity, and a sedentary lifestyle. The final two categories concern two prominent psychosocial situations that have been reliably and repeatedly associated with negative health outcomes: high life stress and low social support.

NONADHERENCE: BASIC PRINCIPLES

Many physicians assume that problems of nonadherence remain largely outside the physician's control and that all that can be done is to give clear advice and just hope the advice will be followed. This is not the case. The interested physician can accomplish a great deal through systematic attention to increasing adherence.

As already mentioned in Chapter 5, the problem of nonadherence is considerable. A large number of patients do not follow advice consistently, and many patients do not follow advice at all. This problem leads to a massive amount of unnecessary suffering and premature death, not to mention wasted resources. The medical profession, as a whole, has only just started to address this problem systematically.[1,2]

This section of the chapter presents five basic principles to guide the physician in addressing the problems of nonadherence to treatment recommendations.

1. Understand the four *intrinsic* factors associated with increased medication adherence.

2. Understand the four *extrinsic* factors associated with increased medication adherence.
3. Accept that physicians will not be able to help or change everyone.
4. Take a long-term view.
5. Understand and use the transtheoretical model of change.

Understanding Four Intrinsic Characteristics of the Medication Regimen that Are Associated with Increased Adherence

Adherence depends partly on the intrinsic character of the regimen. The intrinsic factors that have been shown to increase adherence are consistent with commonsense expectations:

1. Simple regimen
2. Short duration of regimen
3. Obvious positive effects (that is, the patient feels better each time he or she follows the regimen)
4. Few negative effects (e.g., cost, side effects, lifestyle disruption, or other distress)

Sadly, most regimens, if they are to be ethical and effective, and particularly if they involve a change of lifestyle, do not have these characteristics.

Understanding Four Extrinsic (Educational and Motivational) Factors Associated with Increased Adherence to Medication

The way in which the physician approaches the task of education and motivation makes a considerable difference to ultimate adherence, even if the regimen itself is complex, long, and unpleasant.[2] Educational and motivational factors are extrinsic to the character of the regimen. Physicians who attend to the four extrinsic factors described below can expect to increase their patients' adherence to management plans.

1. The presentation of the regimen to the patient emphasizes its compatibility with the patient's own beliefs and expectations.
2. The regimen and the rationale are clearly understood by the patient.
3. The patient has been actively involved in negotiating and choosing the regimen.
4. Adherence is monitored and reinforced by the physician or the patient's significant others.

Accepting the Reality that Physicians Can't Help or Change Everyone

Physicians must accept the reality that they cannot help everyone with lifestyle or other adherence problems. Many of these problems represent long-standing, deeply ingrained behaviors that are refractory to change. For example, many smokers and drinkers may never be able cut down on their substance dependence, regardless of the health benefits of doing so. Physicians must realize that many of their patients can change, but that some may not be able to change. This realization helps prevent the frustration and sense of global hopelessness that can result from a few difficult, treatment-refractory patients.

The realization that some patients cannot change should not become an excuse for nihilism or pessimism. Many, perhaps most, patients with substance abuse or other lifestyle and adherence problems can be helped, especially with physicians' skillful and focused interventions. The pragmatic and targeted suggestions described in this chapter are consistent with the busy practice of general medicine.

Taking a Long-Term View

Patterns of success and failure and progress and relapse characterize lifestyle and related adherence problems.[3] Because they reflect deeply ingrained habits, patients often move forward and backward in repeated cycles of change. These patterns should be expected. Relapse and relapse prevention should be part of patient-physician planning and should not lead to unreasonable patient or physician disappointment.

In addition to accepting that he or she cannot help everyone, the physician must understand that the management of patients with lifestyle problems requires the careful building of a partnership and a long-term plan of action.

Understanding and Using the Transtheoretical Model of Change

Based on observations of the experiences of actual patients, Prochaska and DiClemente[3] proposed a transtheoretical model of change, which has become the most influential conceptual and pragmatic framework for helping patients with lifestyle and related adherence problems.[4] The model has been termed "transtheoretical" because it describes actual observations and is not grounded in the psychologic assumptions of any particular school of thought. It is, in fact, compatible with any of the predominant psychologic theories.

The transtheoretical model both describes patterns of change and suggests appropriate interventions for physicians who want to help their patients change. In brief, patients do not move simply from a state or condition of nonadherence to one of adherence. Typically, individuals who manage to change their behavior proceed through four distinct stages (precontemplation, contemplation, action, and maintenance). When relapse occurs, different versions of the cycle may repeat itself.

The physician who wants to help the patient most effectively must not adopt a "one-size-fits-all" approach. Rather, the physician must determine at which of the four stages the patient resides. The most efficient and powerful behavior change interventions follow directly from an assessment of the patient's stage of readiness for change.

For example, the patient in the stage of *precontemplation* has not even started to think about changing. When the patient starts to think about whether to change, he or she is said to be in the stage of *contemplation*. The stage of *action* begins when the patient begins to do something to change, and *maintenance* involves action to maintain the change and prevent relapse.

For the patient in the stage of precontemplation, the physician's goal should focus on moving the patient from precontemplation to the stage of contemplation. It is generally too ambitious a goal to expect the patient to move from precontemplation directly to action or change. For example, the physician might ask a patient who is drinking too much whether he or she might begin seriously thinking about cutting down. As a motivational intervention, the physician could ask whether the patient's current drinking pattern is perhaps interfering with anything else the patient might want in life (e.g., health, job success, or family relationships).[5] Initiating a discussion that can start the patient really thinking about change should be considered a success, in and of itself.

For a patient at another, more advanced, stage—already contemplating change—the goal of the physician should become helping the patient develop an action plan. For example, the physician can praise the patient for considering change and ask him or her to suggest pragmatic next steps.

Physician: I am really delighted that you are now thinking about cutting down on your drinking. Are you ready to suggest some specific action that could move you forward in this direction?

In sum, physicians who reach an understanding with patients about where they stand in the cycle of change can focus their efforts selectively and will be less likely to become frustrated and more likely to be of help in the long run.

MEDICATION NONADHERENCE

Between 23% and 45% of medical patients do not take their medication as prescribed by their physicians.[1] This can be a frustrating part of the practice of medicine. Physicians who work hard to diagnose and treat their patients may feel confused and bitter when their patients do not follow their advice.

As discussed in Chapter 5, the physician should evaluate the extent of nonadherence in as nonthreatening and accepting a manner as possible. The physician might begin this inquiry in the following manner:

Physician: Most people have great difficulty taking medications exactly as prescribed. What difficulties have you been having?

The physician should offer understanding and legitimation when the patient explains adherence difficulties, and the physician should offer praise for any successes. For example:

Physician: It's good that you're taking the pills as often as you are. I realize it's an inconvenience, and I understand why you skip taking the water pill sometimes during the day because it makes you go to the bathroom too much.

Because many patients do not understand the medication regimen that is prescribed by the physician, it is important to check the patient's understanding of the regimen and of the rationale. The physician can say something such as the following:

Physician: I just want to make sure that we understand each other about the medication schedule. Could you tell me your understanding of the medication plan?
and later
Could you now review your understanding of the reasons why the medication is important?

After the physician has ascertained the extent of the nonadherence and the reasons for it, a modified treatment plan or a renewed contract for adherence to the old one can be negotiated. One way to approach this might be the following:

Physician: Well, I understand it really has been very difficult to stick to the plan. What would you like to do from here? What ideas do you have that might help you? Is there any way that I can be of help to you?

Chapter 5 goes into more detail about the ways the physician can help a patient develop and commit to a treatment plan. In brief, after a suitable plan is developed cooperatively between the patient and the physician, it is essential that the physician schedule frequent and regular follow-up visits to maintain adherence and to prevent relapse. Several excellent books and articles are available that discuss the problem of medication nonadherence in detail.[1,2,4]

LIFESTYLE PROBLEMS

The term "lifestyle" refers to long-term behavioral habits such as smoking, drinking, overeating, and sedentary lifestyle. People find these habits difficult to change, not only because they may be truly substance dependent and therefore subject to withdrawal symptoms, but also because the habit may be genetically determined (in part) or have become part of their self-image.

Alcohol and Substance Abuse and Dependence

Communication with patients who abuse alcohol or drugs is problematic for many reasons. The first problem may be a negative attitude by the physician. Patients with chemical dependency are often seen as weak individuals who are responsible for their own problems and, in any case, are assumed to be resistant to treatment. Physicians with such attitudes will feel little incentive to tackle or even look for alcohol and drug abuse problems.[6] Chemical dependency shares the characteristics of other chronic physical illnesses, and evidence has shown that it is equally treatable when approached properly and systematically.[7-10] Not everyone can fully recover without relapse or recurrence, as is the case for patients with other chronic illnesses. Patients must agree to participate in the treatment program, of course, but many do recover and sustain their recovery over long periods.[7-10]

In communicating with patients who abuse alcohol, as with all patients, the first priority is to build a good relationship. Because alcohol is a sensitive issue, it can be difficult to achieve a relationship that not only feels positive but also includes openness and honesty by both parties. Alcohol abuse is often associated with painful emotions such as guilt, anxiety, and depression. Most patients with alcohol problems are trying to cope as best they can, and even those who deny that drinking is a problem are often already trying to limit their use of it. Proper assessment and effective treatment are possible only if the physician is careful to show consistent empathy for the patients' problems and respect for their efforts to cope.

Recognition is a major problem in the treatment of alcohol-related problems. Perhaps 20% of American men will, at one point in life, meet diagnostic criteria for alcohol abuse,[8] yet only one in five of them ever discusses the problem with a physician.[9] One of the reasons that proper exploration of alcohol issues is so often neglected may be physician anxiety and reluctance to upset a friendly relationship.

Another barrier to recognition is patient denial. The frequency of this problem underscores the need for physicians to pay specific attention to, and sometimes experience, specialized training in the area of alcohol detection.[6] Physicians should not ask patients, "Do you have a problem with alcohol?" When asked in this form, patients will almost always deny the problem, often because they genuinely do not see it in those terms. A better approach is the CAGE interview, reviewed in Chapter 12.

Even if the first interview function (building the relationship) and the second (assessing the problems) are handled well, the third function (managing the problems) still presents special challenges. The patient's beliefs and expectations about his or her use of alcohol have to be carefully explored and respected. Then the physician must find a way to educate the patient that is acceptable and nonthreatening but at the same time honest, clear, and realistic. For example, confronting a patient about the dangers of "creeping" alcoholism is often important.[9] A nonjudgmental way to do this might be something like this:

Physician: I think alcohol might be sneaking up on you without your realizing it.

Obtaining the patient's commitment to a realistic plan for gaining control will usually require carefully exploring the patient's own ideas before negotiating the final agreement. Physicians also need to familiarize themselves with referral sources and local agencies that are available for their patients, such as the local chapters of Alcoholics Anonymous (AA).

Communicating with patients who abuse drugs demands strategies and skills that are much the same as those needed for alcohol, but with additional challenges. Patients who abuse opiates may use physical problems as a vehicle to obtain prescription drugs. Differentiating malingering in the service of chemical dependency from true somatization can be difficult. The best approach is to minimize the use of strong analgesics and follow such patients closely over time to get to know them better.

Consultation with colleagues and experts when necessary (e.g., psychiatrists and psychologists) may prove invaluable. Physicians must be aware of the dangers of iatrogenic abuse of sedative-hypnotics and analgesics. Some patients do indeed need to use habituating medications for their psychiatric or physical disorders. When questions arise as to the true "necessity" of these medications, physicians should make liberal use of consultation with specialist colleagues for the protection of their patients as well as for ethical and medicolegal protection.

Smoking

Cigarette smoking is one of the major self-inflicted health hazards in contemporary society. It has been implicated in the etiology of lung cancer, coronary heart disease, strokes, chronic obstructive lung disease, chronic bronchitis, and many more illnesses.[4] Physicians should do everything they can to help smokers stop or decrease this dangerous habit. Cutting down even in small amounts has been shown to have clear health benefits.

As with any other health issue, the success of the physician's intervention will depend largely on the quality of the relationship he or she has managed to build with the patient. Most smokers today are well aware that the habit is dangerous, so it is obvious that helping them requires much more than just giving didactic information and advice.

In most instances, smoking is a deeply ingrained, habit-forming part of the patient's lifestyle and self-concept and usually also involves true physiologic addiction. Denial, in the psychologic sense, presents a common issue in the treatment of smoking, just as it does in the treatment of alcohol and other substance abuse or dependence. Through the process of denial and rationalization many smokers come to believe either that they are immune to the health risks or that the risks are too insignificant to bother with. Denial is rarely complete, however. Many smokers have tried to limit or stop their habit and may feel embarrassed or guilty about their failure to do so. Physicians who, in their relationship building, demonstrate understanding and respect for these realities of the smokers' situations are more likely to make an impact during the educational component of the interview.

Effective strategies for the education of patients who smoke will use the general principles for lifestyle modification described previously. The following sequence of interventions has been derived from empirical research and should be part of each physician's repertoire[11]:

1. Explore the patient's knowledge and fill in gaps.
2. Explore the patient's intentions and ask "when" if they are interested in thinking about stopping (if they are in the stage of precomptemplation).
3. If patients are in the stage of contemplation, ask if they want to develop a plan to stop.
4. Offer to help patients cut down or stop.
5. Elicit the patient's ideas about strategies.
6. Negotiate a contract.
7. Offer nicotine patches, gum, or bupropion for patients who suffer withdrawal.
8. Provide close follow-up.
9. Expect a relapse and be prepared to renegotiate the contract.
10. Refer interested patients to specialist smoking cessation services.

For physicians interested in developing their own skills in this important area of behavioral interventions with their patients, other readings and workshops are available.[4]

Obesity

Like cigarette smoking, overeating and obesity are well-recognized health hazards. Patients should be offered help in the same way that smokers are approached. Education, offers to help, collaborative negotiation of intervention strategies, and close follow-up are all helpful in the physician's approach to this difficult problem. Patients should be referred to other sources of help (e.g., self-help groups, other agencies, and other professionals) when appropriate.[12]

Sedentary Lifestyle

A sedentary lifestyle has been shown to be related to negative health outcomes. To help motivate patients get more exercise, physicians should follow the strategies discussed previously (e.g., education, elicitation of ideas, contract negotiations, and close follow-up).[4]

PSYCHOSOCIAL RISK FACTORS: HIGH LIFE STRESS AND LOW SOCIAL SUPPORT

High Life Stress

High life stress is not typically regarded as a lifestyle issue that requires physicians to make health-related interventions. However, it is listed here because a considerable amount of data indicates that high life stress, usually as measured by frequent life events (especially negatively valued events such as deaths and other losses), is associated with increased vulnerability to new illnesses, injuries, and accidents, as well as to exacerbations or poor outcomes of previously existing conditions.[13-15]

Physicians may be able to help patients who suffer the health consequences of high life stress. Stress is sometimes caused by events entirely beyond the patient's control. Some events are part of unavoidable developmental transitions (e.g., adolescence, college, childbearing, and retirement). However, some life stresses and changes may be modifiable. Patients experiencing significant life change can be counseled to avoid any unnecessary life changes, at least in the short term. In general, it may not be a good idea to add new changes to a life situation already affected by many other recent life changes.

Physicians may also help patients undergoing life stress by suggesting that they seek outside sources of support, to serve as a buffer against the impact of life changes. Support may come from such efforts as increasing contact with friends and family, contacting self-help groups, or seeking formal counseling.

Some patients who experience a high degree of life change may play a role themselves in these stresses. Such patients may have internal emotional conflicts or personality problems leading to instability in their interpersonal relationships. If a patient's stress indicates a chronic style of life adaptation, the physician alone may not be able to offer much help; however, awareness of the problem, itself, may help. In such circumstances the physician could let the patient know that chronic life stress, or life change, may represent a health hazard. The physician could suggest that the patient try to find ways to decrease the constant life stress and change. Self-help groups, meditation, relaxation training, stress management courses, and formal psychotherapy may all be of considerable assistance to such patients.

To begin working with a patient with high life stress, a physician might say something like the following:

> **Physician:** I am struck by the number of changes and other stresses in your life. It is important for you to realize that such stress levels are likely to affect your health. What thoughts do you have about ways to reduce your life stress?

Low Social Support

Low social support has been shown to predict poor health and even death as an independent variable, even when controlling for all other known risk factors such as prior health, visits to the doctor, life stress, and smoking.[16] There is some controversy about whether the most important support variable concerns some relatively objective measure, such as frequency of contacts with friends or relatives, or whether more subjective measures such as "perceived social support" and "adequacy of support" are more robust health predictors. Regardless of this controversy, low social support in general predicts poor health outcomes.[17]

Knowledge of the significant social-support variable should have some effect on the way physicians practice medicine. Inquiry about current social supports and perceived adequacy of these supports should be part of the evaluation of all patients. A physician might say something like this:

> **Physician:** Now I would like to check on your sources of support. I do this because it is known that personal support contributes to your health. For example, I would like to know—whom can you rely on in a crisis?
>
> *or*
>
> Who can you confide in if you have serious personal or private worries?
>
> *or*
>
> How do you feel about the amount of personal support available to you?

Patients who have low levels of support or who perceive themselves as needing more support than they currently have can be helped by their physicians in several ways. Such patients can be encouraged to begin cultivating more support from friends and family. Sometimes the internal psychologic problems of patients make these efforts problematic. For such patients, formal psychotherapy may be of singular assistance. Other patients can be referred to local self-help groups, informal support groups, and other clubs through which social bonds can be developed.

It is also clear that physician support can become a key variable in many patients' lives. Of course, physicians cannot become friends of patients, but when regular follow-up visits are scheduled, the patient can look forward to this important source of support, especially if the physician allows for at least a few moments of personal time.

Research at the University of Alabama in Birmingham indicated that most patients wanted their physicians to spend some time talking about their personal lives. When this personal discussion occurred, the patients were in general more satisfied. The actual time spent in personal discussion was generally small, often shorter than 5 minutes and almost always shorter than 10 minutes. Yet in more than 90% of cases, patients found this small amount of time sufficient.[18] In encouraging a patient to seek help from family or friends, the physician might say something like this:

> **Physician:** Let's talk about ways to increase the amount of personal support available to you. I feel this could be important for your health. One way that patients do this is by directly telling friends or relatives that they feel a need to talk about special concerns. This can feel awkward because fears of being rejected or of being a burden, but patients usually are surprised by the helpful responses they receive. Do you think this is something you could do?

With respect to seeking support from self-help groups a physician might say something like this:

> **Physician:** Another thing many patients find helpful is to join a self-help group with people who have similar difficulties (e.g., diabetic association, multiple sclerosis association, or grieving widows). Do you think this is something you could do?

The physician can also offer to help the patient himself or herself by saying something like this:

> **Physician:** I would like to be a personal support to you as well. Of course, as your doctor I can't be the same as a friend, but I do want you to know that I am concerned for you as a person as well as wishing to give you good medical advice. I would like to see you regularly, perhaps once a month, to follow your medical problems and try to help you cope with them.

REFERENCES

1. Sackett DL, Snow JC: The magnitude of compliance and noncompliance. In Haynes R, Taylor D, Sackett DL, editors: *Compliance in health care,* Baltimore, 1979, Johns Hopkins University Press.
2. Meichenbaum D, Turk DC: *Facilitating treatment adherence,* New York, 1987, Plenum Press.
3. Prochaska JO, DiClemente CC: Towards a comprehensive model of change. In Miller WR, Heather N, editors: *Treating addictive behaviors: processes of change,* New York, 1986, Plenum Press.
4. Goldstein M et al: Behavioral medicine strategies for medical patients. In Stoudemire A, editor: *Clinical psychiatry for medical students,* Philadelphia, 1990, JB Lippincott.
5. Miller WR, Rollnick S: *Motivational interviewing: preparing people to change addictive behavior,* New York, 1991, Guilford Press.
6. Clark W: Effective interviewing and intervention for alcohol problems. In Lipkin M Jr, Putnam S, Lazare A, editors: *The medical interview: clinical care, research, and education,* New York, 1995, Springer-Verlag.
7. Drummond D, Thom B, Brown C, et al: Specialist versus general practitioner treatment of problem drinkers, *Lancet* 336:915-918, 1990.
8. Finney J, Moos R: The long term course of treated alcoholism. I. mortality, relapse and remission rates and comparison with community controls, *J Stud Alcohol* 52:44-54, 1991.
9. Clark WD, McIntyre JR: The generalist and alcoholism: dilemmas and progress. In Noble J, editor: *Textbook of general medicine and primary care,* ed 3, St Louis, Mosby, in press.
10. Walsh DC et al: A randomized trial of treatment options for alcohol abusing workers, *N Engl J Med* 325:775-782, 1991.
11. Prochaska JO, Goldstein MG: Process of smoking cessation: implications for physicians, *Clin Chest Med* 12:727-735, 1991.
12. Anderson DA, Wadden TA: Treating the obese patient: suggestions for primary care practice, *Archives Fam Med* 8(2)156-167, 1999.
13. Cole S, Saravay S, Levinson R: The biopsychosocial model in medical practice. In Stoudemire A, editor: *An introduction to human behavior,* ed 3, Philadelphia, 1996, JB Lippincott.
14. Cohen SC, Tyrell DJ, Smith AP: Psychological stress and susceptibility to the common cold, *N Engl J Med* 325(9):606-612, 1991.
15. Sarasow IG, Sarsow BR, Potter EH III, et al: Life events, social support, and illness, *Psychosom Med* 47:156, 1985.
16. Berkman LF: The role of social relations in health promotion, *Psychosom Med* 57:245-254, 1995.
17. Seeman TE, Berkman LF, Blazer D, et al: Social ties and support and neuroendocrine function: the MacArthur studies of successful aging, *Ann Behav Med* 16:95-106, 1994.
18. Cohen-Cole SA, Boker J, Bird J, Freeman A: Psychiatric education for primary care: a pilot study of needs, *J Med Educ* 57:931-936, 1982.

CHAPTER

23 Psychosis, Delirium, and Dementia

Psychotic patients and patients with significant cognitive impairment (delirium or dementia) present special and often frightening challenges for the interviewer. Patients with these severe mental disorders represent common problems on inpatient medical services. Understanding general presenting characteristics, inner conflicts and needs, stresses of illness and illness behavior, and interviewing strategies can help physicians deliver better and more efficient care.[1]

PSYCHOTIC PATIENTS

General Characteristics

Psychotic patients have an impairment of their reality-testing abilities or a gross inability to communicate effectively. Psychotic patients generally suffer from hallucinations (sensory perceptions that are not perceived by others, such as hearing voices or seeing visions) or delusions (false beliefs). They may suffer from a gross impairment in the ability to concentrate, think coherently, or communicate effectively.

Inner Conflicts and Needs

Because psychosis has many different manifestations, it is not possible to describe a single set of inner conflicts and needs that uniformly result in psychotic behavior. Furthermore, psychiatrists now believe that most psychotic processes arise from a biologic malfunction of normal integrating circuits in the brain. Although psychologic, social, or physical stresses may provoke or exacerbate a psychotic process, psychotic patients, in general, should be considered as suffering from a brain malfunction.

It can be helpful to view the psychotic patient as struggling to make sense of a bewildering flood of internal and external stimuli. The patient has difficulty making sense of hallucinations, frightening beliefs, or an impaired ability to think coherently. The psychotic patient is usually a frightened patient. He or she can benefit from the physician's help in managing this fear and in managing the flood of internal and external stimuli.

Stresses of Illness and Illness Behavior

The stress of illness itself often precipitates psychosis. A physical insult may be the final common pathway leading to disorganization in psychic functioning. A patient who is already psychotic before the development of a physical illness may become more disorganized because of the stresses and fears of the illness. However, some chronically psychotic patients actually improve mentally when faced with physical stress. This is difficult to understand but is a well-recognized phenomenon.

Psychosis is frightening for patients but also frightening for physicians. While many physicians can empathize with the experience of patients who are anxious, sad, or angry, some are unable to feel anything but fear when faced with psychosis in their patients. Patients who accuse the doctor of poisoning them or who report hearing voices commanding them to kill someone understandably make physicians quite anxious. Patients whose thought processes are so disorganized that they cannot complete sensible sentences also may be intimidating.

Interviewing Strategies

The first principle of interviewing a psychotic patient is to try to remain calm and refrain from panicking. If the patient is threatening, the physician must find some excuse to leave the room immediately and summon security assistance. Physicians should not attempt to be brave or to assume risks. Excellent sources are available for further learning in this area.[2,3]

The physician can help the patient gain control by structuring the interview around simple, nonthreatening questions. The physician should ask the patient to give simple information such as his or her complete name, birth date, and educational history. Open-ended questioning can provoke anxiety. If the patient is afraid, anxious, or angry, the physician can reflect and legitimate these emotions as he or she would with any other patient who is struggling with emotional experiences. Even the angry, paranoid patient can have his or her experience legitimated without the delusion itself being supported. For example:

Physician: I can certainly understand why you would feel so upset because you think you are being poisoned.

The patient may challenge the physician by saying something such as the following:

Patient: Don't you believe me?

The physician should not argue when challenged in this way by a paranoid patient, but neither should he or she support the delusion in any way. A middle path that defers judgment is recommended:

> **Physician:** You ask if I believe you about whether you are being poisoned. I can tell you for sure that I am not poisoning you. I can't tell you for sure right now whether anyone else may be poisoning you, but I'm willing to listen to you and help you in any way I can.

DELIRIOUS OR DEMENTED PATIENTS

General Characteristics

Delirium is a disorder of consciousness in which the ability to interact meaningfully with the environment is compromised because of some brain dysfunction.[4] Delirious patients often become more confused and agitated in the evenings, a condition known informally as "sundowning" (i.e., the exacerbation of confusion in the hours when the sun goes down). Such patients are usually disoriented and unable to carry on a meaningful conversation. At times, this condition can be misdiagnosed as an acute psychotic illness like schizophrenia.

Dementia is the loss of previously acquired intellectual function.[4] Patients with dementia may be able to have a meaningful conversation, but they have lost previously acquired cognitive abilities, most typically memory function.

Inner Conflicts and Needs

The patient with delirium or dementia may feel great distress at the loss of cognitive function. The patient struggles to make sense of the world with diminished or diminishing cognitive resources and may be frightened by his or her lack of understanding. The greatest need may be for an increased sense of understanding and cognitive mastery. Achieving this may not be possible.

Interestingly, some patients with dementia either are unaware of deficits or successfully deny an awareness of these deficits to themselves. Such patients seem quite content despite their deficits.

Stresses of Illness and Illness Behavior

The stress of illness may itself provoke delirium in patients who have compromised mental function (e.g., dementia). The physical stress may be the chief insult, but a change in environment with uncertain procedures and unfamiliar people also may contribute to cognitive disorganization. The illness behavior may be manifested as insatiable demands for information that cannot be adequately supplied. Paranoia and visual hallucinations are also common manifestations of delirium and dementia.

Interviewing Strategies

As with the psychotic patient, the interviewing behaviors that work best for patients with delirium or dementia vary. When emotions such as fear, sadness, or anger present themselves, the same principles of responding to emotions with reflective and legitimating comments can be helpful. Open-ended questions can also provoke anxiety in patients who have limited cognitive capacities. Closed-ended questions about nonthreatening issues are better. Furthermore, reassurance can be helpful. Patients with a new delirium can usually be told something such as the following:

> **Physician:** I am aware that you are having some trouble with confusion right now. This is common in the hospital for patients with illnesses like yours. I expect that you will begin to think more clearly in a few days.

Patients with an irreversible dementia who are also upset about their condition can only be told something like the following:

> **Physician:** I can understand your distress about your memory loss. You do have some memory problem and although there is not a lot I can do to improve it, I can work with you to help you find ways to cope with it better.

CONCLUSION

Patients who have psychosis, delirium, or dementia commonly create anxiety or distress among all caregivers, and especially among student physicians. Reliance on the basic principles of the three-function model can be helpful. However, understanding the source of the anxiety with psychotic and cognitively impaired patients can help interviewers rely less on open-ended questioning (which can increase these patients' anxiety) and more on brief, closed-ended, nonstressful questioning, along with considerable reassurance.

REFERENCES

1. Mance R, Cohen-Cole S: Interviewing the psychotic patient. In Lipkin M Jr, Putnam SM, Lazare A, editors: *The medical interview: clinical care, education, and research*, New York, 1995, Springer.
2. Cassem NH: *The Massachusetts General Hospital handbook of general hospital psychiatry*, ed 4, St Louis, 1997, Mosby.
3. Stern TA, Herman JB, Slavin PL: *The Massachusetts General Hospital guide to psychiatry in primary care*, New York, 1998, McGraw-Hill.
4. American Psychiatric Association: *Diagnostic and statistical manual of mental disorders*, ed 4, Washington, DC, 1988, The Association.

CHAPTER

24 Breaking Bad News

Geoffrey H. Gordon

THE THREE FUNCTIONS AND BREAKING BAD NEWS

In most medical situations the three functions of the interview can be applied in a relatively straightforward, chronologic sequence. The physician can start by building a relationship in which patients feel understood, respected, and supported. Next, the physician can identify and assess patients' problems and concerns. Finally, the physician can manage the problems by providing information, sharing decision making, and motivating patients to adhere to treatment plans. Although all three functions are applied as needed throughout all interviews, the typical chronology is not followed in situations of breaking bad news. In these challenging and emotionally wrenching situations, the functions overlap and occur simultaneously.

One function in breaking bad news is to give information ("Mr. Jones, the test showed that the lump on your x-ray is a lung cancer. We have time to think about what to do next. I'd like to ask Dr. X to advise us on the best treatment, but I'll still be your main doctor."). At the same time, the doctor must gather data ("What do you already know about lung cancer? What kinds of information would you like to have now? Is there anyone else you'd like to include in these discussions?") and build the relationship ("I can see this news is really hard for you. I'm wondering what you're most concerned about right now."). A growing number of studies demonstrate that breaking bad news without relationship building and support, and without attending to meaning and impact of the news, can severely impair patients' and families' coping and functioning.[1]

Why a chapter on breaking bad news? Students are often surprised to learn that U.S. physicians have avoided the practice, study, and teaching of breaking bad news until the last several decades. For example, the percentage of physicians who tell cancer patients the diagnosis rose from 10% in the 1960s to over 90% in the 1980s.[2] Some of this change reflects increasing public awareness of cancer diagnosis and treatment, greater patient autonomy and self-determination, and greater scrutiny of physician practices. However, physicians then and now are poor predictors of patients' desires for information and involvement in medical care and have consistently underestimated patients' desires to know if they have cancer. Most U.S. patients report feeling less isolated and better able to cope when given information about their medical conditions, even when the news is bad. However, they consistently report that their concerns, feelings, and questions are not adequately addressed. We still have a lot to learn about breaking bad news.[3]

Breaking bad news is challenging for patients and physicians. For patients, bad news can mean the threat of multiple losses associated with serious illness, including the possible loss of life. For physicians, breaking bad news can mean acknowledging feelings of helplessness, sadness, or fears of death. From a practical standpoint, carefully orchestrated plans to break bad news can be derailed by other crises or the need to break the news can arise unpredictably, when the time does not feel right or adequate. In addition, neither doctor nor patient knows quite what to expect from the other during the interaction, and this tension and uncertainty can lead either party to end the interaction without proper closure. These challenges inhibit the teaching and learning, as well as the practice, of breaking bad news.

Most of the published literature on breaking bad news is focused on giving the diagnosis of cancer to patients and their families.[4] This chapter draws on that literature and on a few studies of giving parents the news of a child's developmental disabilities, giving the news of a positive test result for the human immunodeficiency virus, and notifying survivors of a loved one's death.

Preparing to Break Bad News

Preparing patients for bad news can begin early in the workup if objective data strongly suggest a serious disorder:

Physician: Mr. Virchow, the blood in your stool and your low blood count really worry me. A lot of things can cause this. Sometimes it's hemorrhoids, which are blood vessels in the rectum. Sometimes it's blood vessels higher up. Sometimes it's polyps, or little growths on the wall of your intestine. These can bleed, and if they've been there a long time, they can even turn into cancer. I think we should do some more tests to find out exactly what it is.

Patient: Really? What kind of cancer, Doc?

Physician: I'm not sure that's what it is. Like I said, we need some more tests. The most important test is to look up inside you and check for anything abnormal. If we see something, we can take out a little piece of it and then tell you what it is. How does that sound to you?

Patient: Well, if that's what you have to do, I guess it's OK.

This is a good opportunity to ask patients how they would like to receive results:

Physician: Whatever we find, we're going to have to talk about what to do next. Is there someone you'd like to come with you to that visit?

Patient: Yeah, my wife. She always wants to know what the doctor says.

Ideally, the primary care physician collects these data and discusses them with the patient and family. In many settings, however, consultants discuss findings with patients and arrange follow-up care. At the very least, primary care physicians can stay in the information loop and provide some continuity, if not coordination, of care around the breaking of bad news.

The physician's preparation must include a clear understanding of the diagnosis, possible treatment options, a general idea of prognosis, and specific plans for what will happen next in the way of consultations, tests, and return visits. Preparation should include setting aside adequate time for the task and assessing the physician's own feelings about the news (addressed in the "Importance of Physician Self-Awareness" section later in this chapter).

Choosing a Setting

Patients report that they prefer to receive bad news from a physician, preferably one who knows them and their medical conditions. Thus it should not be delegated to other health care team members (as is sometimes the case). Finding a private room is difficult in many settings, but breaking bad news while standing in a busy hallway can and should be avoided. Sitting down and making eye contact is an effective way to communicate attention and concern.

Occasionally bad news must be broken at a distance:

Physician: Mrs. Jones? This is Dr. Welby at Mercy General. I'm the doctor on call this evening, and I need to talk with you about your husband's condition. Are you able to come to the hospital?

Mrs. Jones: Is this about Harold?

Physician: Yes it is. I'm afraid his condition has worsened and we'd really like you to come. Do you have a way to get here?

Mrs. Jones: I'll come right away.

Death notification by telephone is sometimes necessary when families ask directly if death has occurred or if they are unable to come to the hospital.

Mrs. Jones: I'll come right away. He isn't dead, is he?

Physician: Yes, I am terribly sorry to have to tell you this over the phone, but I am afraid he has just died. He died peacefully around eight o'clock tonight. Is anyone there with you now?

Mrs. Jones: No, but I can call my sister. She said to call if I need anything. I'm sure she would bring me to the hospital. I hate to lose him, but he was suffering so . . . (sobbing)

Physician: I'd like to see you when you arrive. Please come right up to the seventh floor and ask for Dr. Welby. We can talk some more then.

Attributions and Expectations

Nearly all patients have assumptions about what might be wrong (attributions) and what needs to be done to help them (expectations). Attributions and expectations are based on experiences with self, family, friends, informal health advisors, the media, and other sources. They develop before the medical visit and may play a role in the decision to seek care. They are a context into which the patient will try to fit the physician's explanations and recommendations. To understand the meaning of the illness to the patient, the level of information the patient desires, and the patient's emotional reaction to bad news, the physician must understand the patient's attributions and expectations about the problem.

Physician: Mr. Virchow, I wonder what you've been thinking about this blood in the stool and your low blood count. What do you think is wrong?

Patient: I don't know, Doc. That's why I came to see you.

Physician: I understand that, and I'll tell you what I think, but it often helps me to know what you've already learned about this, or what concerns you the most about it.

Patient: Well, I did see a piece in the paper awhile back that talked about blood in the stool. It was all about colon cancer. They said by the time you find it, it's too late to do anything about it. They said you should eat broccoli.

Physician: What would colon cancer mean to you?

Patient: Well, my mother had some kind of cancer. They opened her up and saw it everywhere and just closed her up again. She died in agony two weeks later.

Physician: OK, let me make sure I understand. You've wondered if this might be colon cancer. And your experience tells you that cancer is painful and fatal. That must be really frightening for you. You did the right thing by coming in and getting checked out. You need to know, though, that if we can find colon cancer early, there's a lot we can do to treat it. We're also much better at treating the symptoms of cancer. Now let me tell you about the biopsy and what we're going to do next.

This patient's prior knowledge and concerns can help the physician anticipate the kinds of information and emotional support the patient will need as bad news is given. Eliciting attributions and expectations is a key step in breaking bad news.

Breaking the Bad News

The first step in breaking bad news is assessing what the patient is ready to hear.[5] The physician usually can do this by reviewing the clinical data, checking the patient's understanding and concerns about the data, and indicating that new information is available:

Physician: Mr. Virchow, you know that we saw a lump on the wall of your intestine and took a biopsy of it. What have you already learned about the results?

Consider these possible responses:

Patient: Well, is it cancer?
Patient: Could you wait till my wife gets here? She gets off work at 6 o'clock.
Patient: (silent, stares at the doctor's face)

Patients who immediately ask if the diagnosis is cancer are ready to hear the news. Others may indicate, verbally or nonverbally, that they are uncomfortable proceeding. For these patients, techniques to slow down the message may be appropriate. Buckman[6] describes the "warning shot," a statement that the condition is more serious than first thought, to assess the patient's readiness to go on. He also describes giving a choice about how to hear the news, something such as: "Are you a sort of person who likes lots of information and detail about your condition, or a sort of person who likes a brief summary and recommendations?" This technique honors patients' individual wishes and styles. Maguire,[7] recognizing that patients remember little of what is said to them after bad news is broken, describes giving the most important message first:

Physician: Whatever I tell you in a moment, I want you to remember, the situation is serious, but there's plenty we can do. We'll have to work closely together over the next several months.

The main danger in slowing down the delivery of bad news is that physicians may fail to deliver (or patients may fail to hear) the message clearly and unambiguously. Most patients favor a direct statement of the news, followed by a pause while the message sinks in, and are then able to respond:

Physician: I'm afraid that the biopsy showed cancer of the colon.
Patient: Oh, my God, doctor. Not cancer (weeps, wrings hands). Oh, my God. What am I going to do now?
Physician: I know this comes as a shock. This wasn't what you were expecting at all. But I want you to know that we'll take it one step at a time and work on it together. The next big step is to find out if it has spread outside the colon. To start that we'll do a CT scan of your belly. That will help us decide on the best treatment.

Emotional Support

Patients who receive bad news usually remember the physician's attitude and manner more vividly than the technical details of the news. Physicians must be able to convey an attitude of honesty and caring even in the face of strong and varied emotions. The greatest challenge for physicians is to remain with patients, accept strong emotional reactions as normal and legitimate responses to bad news, and express support and partnership for the present and future. Dame Cicely Saunders, originator of the hospice movement in the United Kingdom, said, "The real secret is not what you tell your patients, but what you let your patients tell you."

Patients' reactions to bad news are individualized and difficult to predict. Common immediate reactions include shock, disbelief, anger, fear, and grief. Patients shocked by bad news report feeling "stunned" or "dazed" and unable to identify specific thoughts or feelings. These patients are among the most challenging because their ideas and feelings are temporarily inaccessible. The physician should ask shocked patients whom they normally talk with about serious problems (e.g., a close friend, family member, or spiritual counselor) and how they plan to get in touch with that person. The stunned state should be acknowledged and future expressions of feelings legitimized:

Physician: I can see that you're feeling overwhelmed right now. I imagine you're quite stunned by this news and that it is hard to even think about. Have I got it right?
Patient: Yes. I can't believe this is happening. I'm going to wake up in a minute and this will all be a bad dream.
Physician: I wish it were so. Is there anyone that I can call for you? Anyone at home that you can be with?
Patient: Yes, my husband should be home by now.
Physician: You two will probably have some questions or concerns that you'd like to talk about with me. If you'd like, I can call him for

you now and explain what has happened. Then I'd like the two of you to come see me tomorrow afternoon, so we can talk about what to do next.

Disbelief or denial is a normal psychologic response that protects people from being overwhelmed by bad news. Most patients in denial are ambivalent, or "of two minds," about the news. Most doctors have experienced carefully breaking bad news to a patient, only to have the patient respond to someone else's questions with, "They're not sure yet what it is" or, "I think I'm just run down."

A patient who only intermittently acknowledges the bad news upsets family and medical personnel, who expect grief, a discussion of treatment options, informed consent, or advance directives. Buckman[6] notes that at the beginning, denial can help patients cope one step at a time and that arguing, persuading, or "proving" the bad news is counterproductive. Denial later on inhibits rational decision making. The need and capacity for patients to participate in care need to be evaluated further. This evaluation should include assessment of decision-making capacity (e.g., is the patient able to complete a Mini-Mental Status Exam?). Buckman also recommends evaluating insight (does the patient acknowledge denial when it is pointed out?), motivation (does the patient want to change the behavior?), and flexibility (will the patient take steps to modify the behavior?). For example, the patient should be asked to consider what decisions might have to be faced if the condition worsens:

Physician: What kinds of decisions and plans should we make now, in case you're not feeling well enough to make them in the future?

If it is unclear whether a patient's maladaptive denial can be changed, a mental health consultation is indicated.

In the United States in this era of patient autonomy and self-determination, treating a patient who is cognitively intact but cannot demonstrate clear knowledge of the procedure, risks, and alternatives is inadvisable.

Some patients become angry when receiving bad news and direct this anger toward the physician. Physicians experience this as a personal attack and can become defensive or angry in return. A more effective approach is to understand that anger is a normal reaction to bad news and that acknowledging and respecting angry feelings disarms rather than escalates them:

Patient: What do you mean, the cancer is back? I did everything you told me. I took all the treatments and followed all your advice. There's got to be some mistake!

Physician: I've double checked the tests, and I'm sure it's back. This was a surprise to me, too. This isn't what either of us expected. You did all the right things, and now this happens. I can see how you'd be angry.

Patient: (agitated) Why didn't you find it sooner? I could have been cured!

Physician: I know it just doesn't make sense. We followed all the recommended screening procedures and it still happened. Being angry, even with me, is OK. But I'd still like to be your doctor and help you fight this again. Can we talk about that now, or would you like some time to think about it?

Some patients are fearful and grief stricken by bad news. For these patients, empathic statements are particularly useful:

Patient: (trembling and weeping) Don't let this happen to me, please! I've got two kids in grade school! You don't understand—I can't have this cancer back again!

Physician: I can see this is a terrible blow for you, and you're doing everything you can to cope. And I can see that your biggest concern is looking out for your family. I want you to know that I'll still be your doctor and I want to stick with you on this.

Patient: Yes, please don't give up on me! My husband—he doesn't know what the kids need—he won't even be able to handle this himself. What can I tell him?

Physician: (touching her shoulder) Why don't you ask him to come in with you? I know someone who can help the two of you deal with this together and also decide what to tell the kids. We can schedule it for later this week.

Of the possible responses to patients' feelings (a closed-ended question, an open-ended question, giving information, or an empathic statement), empathy is the one most likely to move the interview in a useful direction. Conveying empathy (truly understanding how a patient feels) is different from expressing sympathy (your feelings about the patient or the situation). Empathic communication has a number of key steps (more intensive application of the basic rapport-building interventions).

1. *Signposting,* or forecasting ("Let me make sure I understand.")
2. *Reflection*, or naming the feeling ("You put in your time on months of painful treatments and beat this breast cancer. Now, two years later, you find it is back. And you're really feeling cheated, because you did all the right things to beat it. Have I got it right?")
3. *Legitimation* ("I think anyone would feel the same way.")
4. *Respect* ("I think you're doing the right thing by taking it on again.")

5. *Support* ("I'd like to help you through this.")
6. *Partnership* ("We'll need to work together, just as hard as last time.")

Patients who request a tranquilizer or sleeping pill to dull the feelings associated with bad news should understand that it is normal to be upset or sad and to sleep poorly after receiving bad news. Depending on the severity of the anxiety or sleeplessness, however, judicious use of psychoactive medication may be helpful in supporting adaptation.

Giving Information

In addition to emotional support, most patients want and need information.[8] Patients given the news of a serious cancer often want to know absolutely that the diagnosis is correct, how much the disease has spread, how it can be treated or cured, and what to expect with the various treatment options. As discussed earlier in this chapter, some patients want lots of information and involvement in decision making, whereas others just want a few sentences about diagnosis and treatment. The best method for giving information is to find out first what the patient already knows (see the "Attributions and Expectations" section). This is an opportunity to correct any misconceptions the patient might have and to tailor information to fill in gaps in the patient's understanding.

Even with careful explanations, patients have difficulty understanding or recalling information given along with bad news. Some basic information-giving techniques include using simple, clear words instead of medical jargon, giving small amounts of information at a time, and summarizing periodically. The physician should check patients' understanding by acknowledging that sometimes doctors' explanations can be unclear and by asking them to repeat what they have understood so far. Drawings or simple metaphors are often useful. If preprinted materials are used, they should be personalized by highlighting information relevant to the patient's situation. Patients should also be encouraged to write down questions that come up between visits and bring them in at scheduled appointments. Some physicians make audio tapes of this interview when breaking bad news, so that patients and families can listen more than once to the information they have been given. Some patients learn from and are emotionally supported by other patients who have the same condition and are willing to share their experiences.

Patients may ask tough questions, such as, "Am I going to die?" and, "How long do I have?" These questions deserve direct and honest answers. In all cases, however, patients should be given hope for support and partnership.

Physician: I think what you're asking is whether you will die because of this cancer. There are statistics on how long people with this kind of cancer live, with and without treatment, but they are just averages. Some patients live much longer and some shorter than the average. I can tell you the averages for your condition, but I can't predict how long you have. I want to tell you again that I am here to help and support you through this.

Other patients are less direct, prolonging conversations, interrupting with new questions, or restarting the interview while the physician is trying to close it. These are signs that important but difficult topics still need to be addressed and that the patient may need some help. The following type of comment may be helpful:

Physician: I can see that there is something troubling you, but that it is hard to talk about. I'd like to hear what's on your mind, either now or when you're ready.

When notifying survivors of a loved one's death, a few additional considerations apply. Survivors will often want to see the deceased's body. This is an important part of the grieving process and should not be denied. Survivors are often concerned about whether their loved one was alone at the time of death, if he or she suffered, and if there was anything they could or should have done differently during the events leading up to the death. Finally, survivors should be asked about anatomical gifts such as corneas, skin, or bone. Families may find comfort in making an anatomical gift; however, certain conditions such as malignancy or infection may preclude the possibility of organ donation. Most medical centers now have specially trained personnel who can screen for organ donation eligibility and talk with families about consent for donation.

Closing the Bad News Interview

Before closing the bad news interview, the physician should think about the dual tasks of managing the relationship and exchanging information. If only one has been completed, the physician acknowledges the missing piece to the patient and opens the door to further discussion:

Physician: We've talked about a lot of information today. I'm also wondering how you're feeling about all this. After all, that's another important part of you and your medical care.

The easiest and most effective way to close the bad news interview is to outline specific further steps. This includes asking who else needs to know the news, how the patient plans on telling those individuals, and if the patient wants help telling them. It also involves gathering more information through consultants and diagnostic tests. In a primary care relationship (comprehensive, continuity, coordinated care), the physician should emphasize that consultants and technicians will be temporarily invited into the relationship but that the physician will be the continuity person throughout the entire illness. The patient should leave with a return appointment regardless of whether new tests or consultations will take place in the interim. At each visit, successful coping is reinforced and additional sources of support are identified, if possible. The physician should ensure a continuity of care even if he or she disagrees with the patient's choices of treatment options.

Importance of Physician Self-Awareness

Breaking bad news affects physicians as well as patients. As patients do with physicians, physicians bring personal experiences, values, attitudes, and biases to their interactions with patients. Breaking bad news adds an additional challenge. When there is little treatment to offer, it gives rise to feelings of inadequacy and guilt. When the bad news is life threatening, it challenges physicians' belief in the power of aggressive biotechnology to overcome disease and makes them feel vulnerable to patients' blame. For some physicians a patient's death means a failure of knowledge, responsibility, or dedication.

Some data suggest that physicians fear death and helplessness more than lay persons do. Clearly, physicians' own assumptions and feelings about patients, medicine, and doctoring can affect communication, and physician self-awareness of these characteristics and "hot buttons" can enhance communication.

Many training programs encourage physicians to suppress their emotions for the sake of "objectivity." This suppression is reinforced through intense work schedules and little time to reflect on personal reactions to patient care. Physicians who fear displaying their emotions can appear cold and uncaring to patients when giving bad news. For example, several studies show that parents receiving bad news about a child felt supported when the informant also appeared distressed and offended when the informant was "professional" and detached. The refusal to acknowledge emotions in self and others, combined with poor training in communication and interpersonal skills, leads physicians to withdraw in response to patients' emotional responses to bad news. This withdrawal can lead to burnout, or feelings of personal isolation and disconnection from the work of patient care. Many training programs now include activities that encourage reflection and self-awareness with the goal of improving clinical care and job satisfaction.

Special Challenges in Breaking Bad News

Losing hope is a fearful circumstance for physicians, patients, and families, who feel that it must be avoided at all costs. Patients are most vulnerable to a loss of hope at the time a life-threatening diagnosis is first made, at the time of recurrence after seemingly successful treatment, and at the time of transition from definitive to palliative care. To physicians, hope means cure, remission, or at the very least a treatment response, and these hopes are conveyed explicitly or implicitly to patients. Few physicians have learned how to give bad news in ways that convey positive support, encouragement, and optimism. This can be done in a variety of ways; for example, by using positive words ("Your scan shows that your liver is normal and healthy") instead of negative ones ("Your liver scan is negative").

Illness can also be presented as a challenge to be met with new coping skills, like other challenges the patient has met and coped with in the past. Such skills can include hoping for different things at different times (for example, hoping first for cure, then for best use of time remaining, then for resolving personal conflicts, then finally for an acceptable quality of life and a painless death surrounded by loved ones). Patients can also learn to influence their quality of life through their thoughts, attitudes, and activities (e.g., learning how to find new sources of pleasure and self-esteem).

The "dark side" of never losing hope can be (1) patients feeling that they have failed at being "positive enough" if the illness progresses, (2) loss of opportunities to grieve together or say good-bye, and (3) loss of focus on the goal, which is an improved quality of life rather than reversal of disease.

Some patients specifically request not to be told bad news. They may have misconceptions about the disease or its treatment. Ask patients what the bad news would mean to them, and what they fear might happen if they receive it (see "Attributions and Expectations" and "Giving Information" sections). Explain the rationale for knowing the news:

Patient: Doctor, if the news is bad, I'd just rather not hear it. Do what you have to do, but don't tell me about it.

Physician: If I understand correctly, you're saying that you don't want lots of information and explanations about what we've found and what we're doing. Many people feel that way, and I certainly won't force information on you. Of course, we need your permission to treat you, whether or not you want these explanations and choices. I can put a note in your chart that you preferred that we make these decisions for you.

Patient: What's the point? I'd just rather you treat me and I'll deal with it.

Physician: We can certainly do that. We know, though, that your job here is to create the best environment for our treatments to work. We think your ideas and feelings would help us plan the best treatment. But if we don't know what those are, we have to guess. I think the more you learn about this, the more we can tailor care to fit you individually.

Sometimes family members will ask that a patient not be given bad news. Families should be reassured that information won't be forced on the patient, but also advised that the patient's knowledge of and participation in care will increase its effectiveness. Families may have had unfortunate experiences with bad news in the past, or may have strong cultural beliefs about how bad news should be given and received. In some cultures, for example, bad news is routinely withheld from patients so that they don't worry or grieve. In other cultures, giving bad news is traditionally a family event and everyone must be present when the patient gets the news. It may help to share your dilemma with the patient (e.g., "Your family has told me that you would prefer not to know some important facts about your condition. What are your thoughts about this?"). Cultural consultants in the form of translators or patient advocates can sometimes mediate cultural or ethnic differences around giving bad news, informed consent, and active participation in care.

Many patients with cancer want to participate in nonallopathic as well as traditional Western medical treatment. Resources that explain the procedures, rationale, and risks of alternative and complementary medicine are now available to physicians. The physician should encourage patients to talk about any other care they are receiving so that it will not combine with allopathic treatments and make them worse. Patients may decline usual medical care or drop out of treatment protocols prematurely. If this occurs, establish that they have decision-making capacity and are making an informed decision. Honor the decision even if it seems to reflect poor judgment. The physician can encourage patients to join advocacy, self-help, and peer support groups to learn what has worked for others receiving allopathic treatment.

CONCLUSION

Breaking bad news is receiving the attention it deserves, as research demonstrates the importance of communication skills on health outcomes and as the developed world's population lives long enough to develop chronic and treatable diseases.[9] Giving bad news requires that all three functions of the medical interview be used simultaneously: give information, assess its emotional impact, and gather data to guide the giving of more information. Particular challenges include patients and families who ask that bad news not be given, physicians who lack the attitudes, skills, and self-awareness to give bad news effectively, and both parties when bad news is given without a plan for the future and a sense of hope.

REFERENCES

1. Girgis A, Sanson-Fisher RW: Breaking bad news: consensus guidelines for medical practitioners, *J Clin Oncol* 13:2449-2456, 1995.
2. Tolle SW, Elliot DL, Girard DE: How to manage patient death and care for the bereaved, *Postgrad Med* 78:87-95, 1985.
3. Fallowfield L: Delivering sad or bad news, *Lancet* 341:476-478, 1993.
4. Muller JH, Desmond B: Ethical dilemmas in a cross-cultural context: a Chinese example, *West J Med* 157:323-327, 1992.
5. Brewin TB: Three ways of giving bad news, *Lancet* 337:1207-1209, 1991.
6. Buckman R: *How to break bad news: a guide for health care professionals*, Baltimore, 1992, Johns Hopkins University Press.
7. Maguire P, Faulkner A: Communicating with cancer patients and handling bad news and difficult questions, *BMJ* 297:907-909, 1988.
8. Krahn GL, Hallum A, Kime C: Are there good ways to give bad news? *Pediatrics* 91:578-582, 1993.
9. Quill TE, Townsend P: Bad news: delivery, dialogue, dilemmas, *Arch Intern Med* 151:463-468, 1991.

UNIT VI

HIGHER-ORDER SKILLS

CHAPTER

25 Nonverbal Communication

Cecile A. Carson

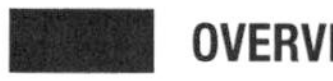

OVERVIEW

Nonverbal communication refers to all behavioral signals that send interpersonal messages and reflect the tenor of interactions between the physician and the patient. Attention to these signals allows the interviewer to monitor the process of an interaction—to keep a finger on the pulse of what transpires in a dynamic, moment-to-moment manner as he or she moves through the three functions of the medical interview. Most important, understanding nonverbal signals allows the interviewer to guide the physician-patient interaction in a positive direction.

Using nonverbal communication effectively does not take extra time, because nonverbal communication occurs in real time, simultaneous with the verbal flow of an interview. Approximately 80% of essential communication between individuals occurs nonverbally, involuntarily, and outside of conscious awareness. Verbal behavior can be deceptive and misleading; people can lie. Nonverbal behavior speaks the truth; in general, nonverbal signals cannot lie. Important information that cannot be hidden is exchanged at all times—from patient to clinician and from clinician to patient. Only 20% of essential communication is verbal and voluntary. Thus the patient and the physician have control over only a small portion of communication. A patient will nonverbally signal any problems he or she has with the three functions of the interview, even if the problem is not expressed verbally. In general, the physician's problems will also be expressed nonverbally outside of conscious awareness.

The four general categories of nonverbal communication are as follows:

1. *Kinesics*—facial expressions, gestures, touch, body tension, position, and angulation
2. *Proxemics*—spatial relationships and barriers
3. *Paralanguage*—voice tone, rhythm, volume, emphasis, and rate of speech

4. *Autonomic output*—flushing, blanching, sweating, tearing, piloerection, changes in breathing and pupil size, swallowing, and dry mouth

BASIC BEHAVIOR

Feeling safe is a basic human need involving self-protection and self-preservation. The patient needs to know if he or she is safe enough with the physician to expose real concerns, fears, and vulnerability.

If the patient does not feel safe, he or she will typically demonstrate behaviors such as fight, flight, or conservation-withdrawal. The alert clinician quickly reads nonverbal behavior and determines whether the patient across the nonverbal space feels safe at any one moment.

Safety

Feelings of safety are reflected by body signals of engagement, relaxation, and a physically open stance. These include low general body tension and the relaxation of facial muscles, with arms and legs relaxed and uncrossed. The patient who feels safe shows more variety in both gestures and voice as the sense of safety gives rise to freer expression.

Fight

The stance of the patient who demonstrates the fight response is most often a stance of engagement and of attack or retaliation as a defense against feeling unsafe. Typical nonverbal signals of a fighting feeling include a forward lean and jutting jaw, clenched fists, and a narrowing of the eyes with inner brows lowered and the mouth tense. The patient may also have a flushed face, flaring nostrils, increased voice volume, and deeper breathing.

Flight

Most of the nonverbal cues demonstrated by a patient experiencing the flight response involve disengagement and withdrawal; the patient leans away, pushes back in a chair, or turns the head down and away. The voice flees as the volume diminishes, the breath flees as it becomes more shallow or is held, and facial color flees (blanching). Other typical cues include putting up physical barriers such as crossed arms and legs and averting the eyes or turning the head away.

Conservation-Withdrawal

Conservation-withdrawal refers to the patient's reaction to feeling overwhelmed with excessive input and to being unable to mount a defensive response. The patient reacts this way when he or she receives unacceptable news, suffers irretrievable loss, or becomes significantly depressed. The patient typically demonstrates a nonverbal pattern of disengagement and relative immobility or quiescence.[1] The patient's body appears slumped rather than relaxed. The patient has a sagging face and slack jaw and slow, shallow breathing. Usually the patient does not appear to use the arms and legs as protective barriers.

> ***It is important to read the overall pattern of nonverbal responses rather than to rely on any one sign. Nonverbal signals should not be oversimplified or overinterpreted.***

Patients sometimes cross their arms and legs because it is cold, because there are no arms to the chair, or as a convention of etiquette, yet their body may be quite relaxed and engaged and their voice melodious, indicating an overall sense of safety in the encounter. Although cultural differences in nonverbal behavior affect comfort levels with interpersonal distance and touch and often will be expressed as a variety of gestures, and eye gazes, nonverbal expressions of safety are universal. Issues of safety in the encounter will show uniformly in the amount of the patient's body tension and autonomic responses and in facial expressions of anger, fear, sadness, surprise, disgust, and joy.[2] Mixed responses such as fight *and* flight are also frequent. A flushed face and loud voice combined with crossed arms or with a turn away from the physician can signal anger at the clinician or the situation and reluctance or fear of overtly expressing the anger.

NONVERBAL SKILLS

Helping the patient move from not feeling safe to feeling safe is crucial to creating a therapeutic milieu in which to gather high-quality information from the patient, assess readiness to change, and negotiate a treatment plan. The skilled physician can use specific nonverbal interventions to facilitate the interview process:

1. Develop nonverbal rapport.
2. Shape the space of the encounter.
3. Address mixed messages.

Developing Nonverbal Rapport

Rapport means "I am with you," and represents the *nonverbal structure of empathy*. Defined as "nonverbal synchrony between two persons," rapport behaviorally consists of two parts, *matching* and *leading*.

Matching is the process of moving as the other person moves, in such a way as to acknowledge aspects of the other person's behavior as a reflection of his or her emotional state. The physician can use any aspect of the patient's behavior: facial expressions, voice volume and rate, body angulation, or gestures. As the physician begins to create synchrony with the patient, he or she begins to enter the patient's world. Patients unconsciously recognize this nonverbal engagement. Their *conscious* recognition is typically through a feeling of being understood by the physician, which can occur even before or without the transmission of verbal information.

The physician must be graceful, respectful, and cautious when matching. Small, gentle efforts at matching should be used; otherwise, the patient may feel manipulated and mocked rather than supported.

The beauty of enhancing rapport nonverbally is that it does not involve extra time, because it occurs simultaneously with the process of gathering verbal information from the patient. However, if rapport is ignored, the patient can feel unsupported if his or her posture and rhythms are not in synchrony with the physician's.[3] Without rapport, the interview will be inefficient and ineffective.

What might matching look like? The confident, compassionate, and skilled physician matches the patient's nonverbal behavior without conscious awareness of what he or she is actually doing. However, understanding the process of matching can increase the interviewer's efficiency and effectiveness. For example, the physician may match a withdrawn patient's posture by leaning forward, with his or her head slightly down and the shoulders drawn slightly inward (Figure 25-1). This facilitates the building of rapport and helps the patient feel understood.

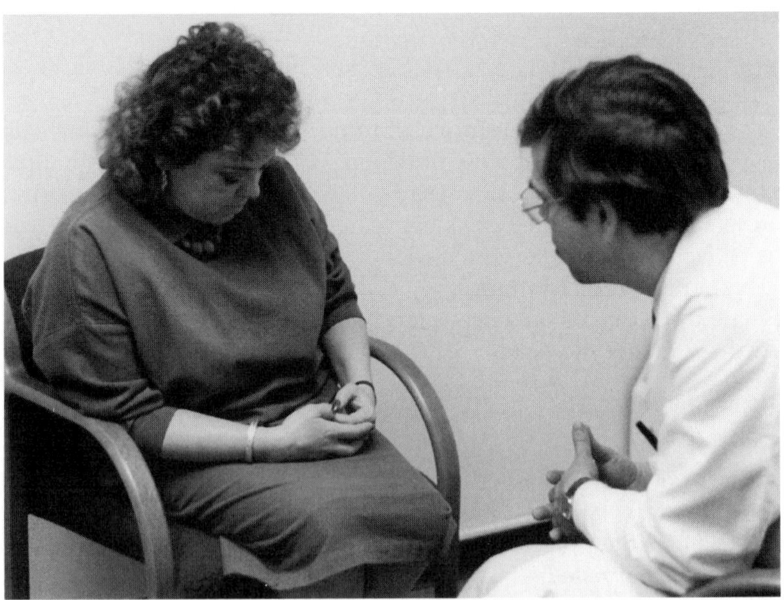

FIG. 25-1 Matching.

A second example is that of a physician who notices rapport problems when facing a highly guarded patient whose arms and legs are crossed tightly and whose body is tense. The cautious physician begins the interaction with his or her own arms (and perhaps legs) loosely crossed, nonverbally acknowledging and accepting the patient's guardedness. The physician performs most of this matching without thinking about it. If the physician leans in too close to the patient, the patient may interpret this as an invasion of personal space and an intrusive response. Even if the physician's intent is to be inviting, the guarded patient may respond to this nonverbal intrusion by withdrawing into an even tighter presentation (Figure 25-2).

Leading refers to the use of the interactional synchrony that has been set up by matching. Patients who feel increased rapport are motivated to try to maintain that feeling; therefore, a leading motion by one person of a pair may produce a reciprocal response by the other person. Leading invites the patient to move with the physician rather than to feel rushed or coerced into responding.

Leading can be a test of whether the interactional synchrony is present. This test consists of making a leading motion within the patient's awareness and observing to see if the patient unconsciously follows the

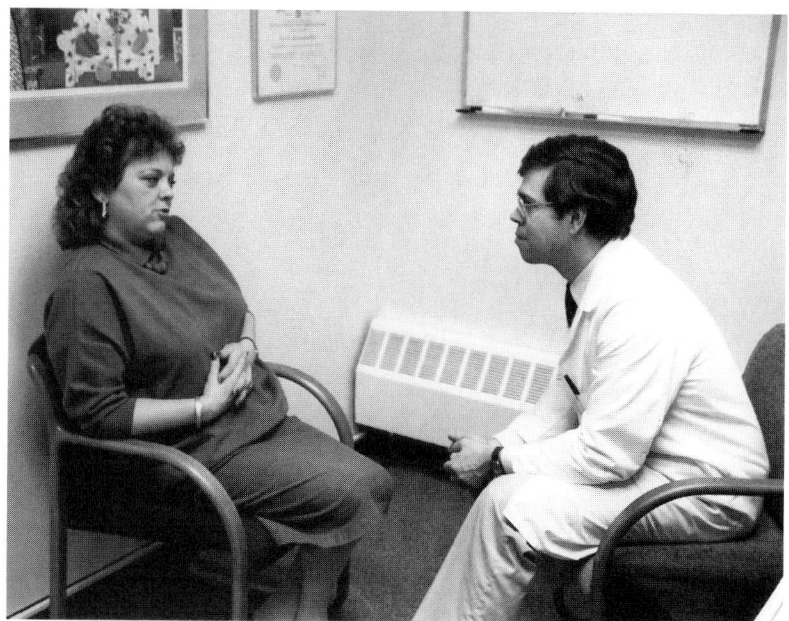

FIG. 25-2 Mismatching.

lead. The physician's leading motion can be a behavioral shift, such as a movement, a gesture, or a change in voice or breathing. Synchrony is present if the patient follows these leading motions. The response to the lead does not have to be an exact duplication; a movement or shift in the general direction of the lead is an adequate indicator. For example, the clinician may reach up and push his or her glasses higher up on the bridge of his nose; the patient may respond quite unknowingly by reaching up immediately afterward and touching his or her own chin.

If the interviewer leads the patient too fast or too dramatically, the rapport will be broken. If the interviewer becomes aware of this break, he or she can recover rapport quickly by returning to matching. Anything new or different that is introduced into the interaction can also be considered leading, either by the provider or by the patient. For example, screening questions about social and sexual history and recommendations such as medication, procedures, and referrals all create something new in the interaction.

Shaping Space

Intentionally shaping the physical space of an encounter sets the form for reflective listening and for the quality of the relationship. How the clinician arranges the spatial relationships in the room frequently parallels how he or she views the interpersonal relationship with the patient. Specific components of the space include the following:

1. The amount of interpersonal distance between people
2. The vertical height differences (such as lying, sitting, and standing)
3. The presence of physical barriers (such as a desk, chair sizes, charts, and bed rails)
4. The angles of facing each other (full face, shoulder-to-shoulder, or angles in between)

Interpersonal distance relates to territoriality. If the clinician is too close during an interview, the patient will feel that his or her space has been encroached on and may try to restore the proper distance (e.g., by looking away, crossing arms or legs to provide a "frontal barrier," flushing, or changing the topic to a less personal one) (Figure 25-3). If the clinician is too far away, true engagement with the patient may be discouraged and a sense of disinterest will be conveyed.

Vertical height differences relate to power. At the start of an encounter, many patients already feel vulnerable and at a disadvantage relative to the clinician. The clinician can help minimize this feeling in the patient by being sensitive to vertical height differences that may exaggerate the patient's disadvantaged position and by being willing to shift his or her position to be at the same level as or below the patient (Figures 25-4 to 25-6).

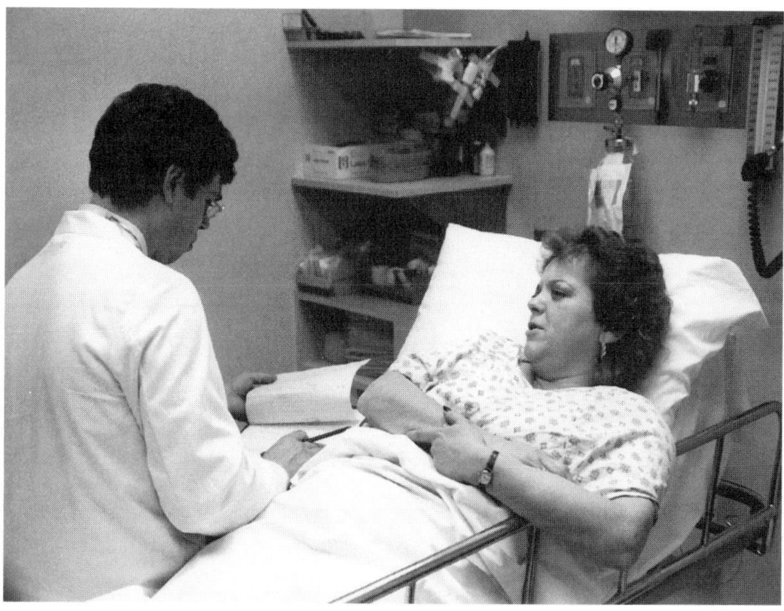

FIG. 25-3 Physician too close to patient.

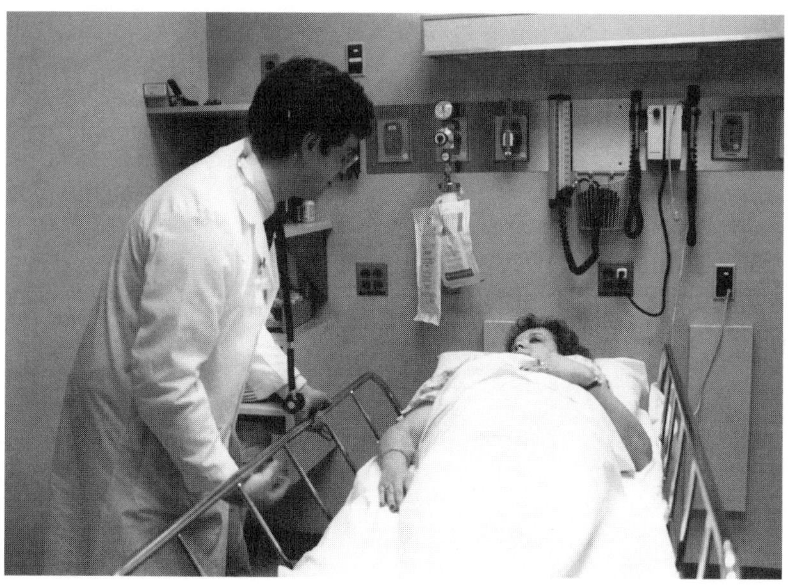

FIG. 25-4 Physician too high.

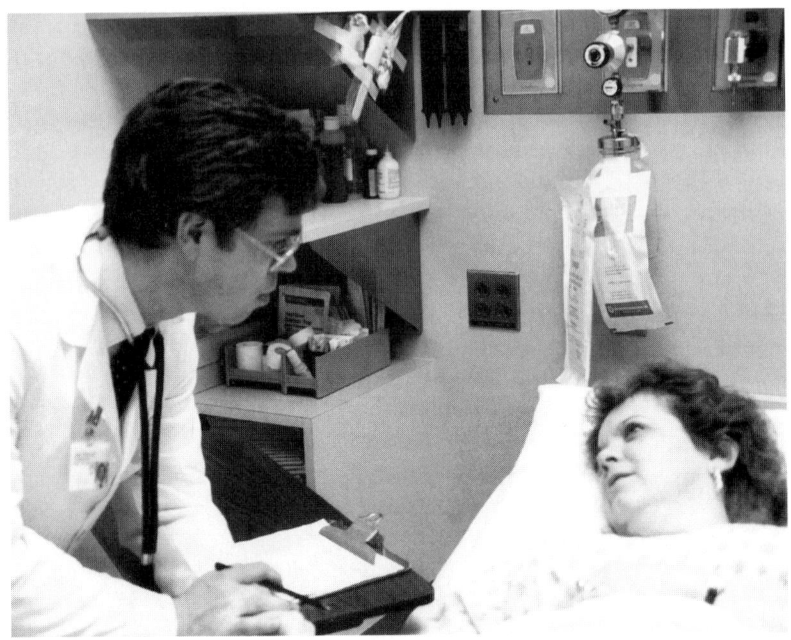

FIG. 25-5 Physician still too high.

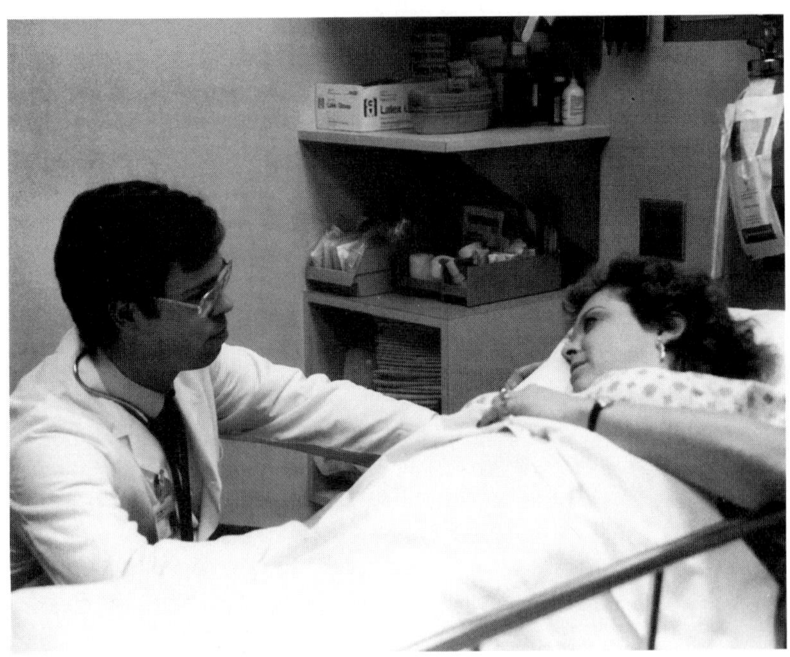

FIG. 25-6 Vertical height equal.

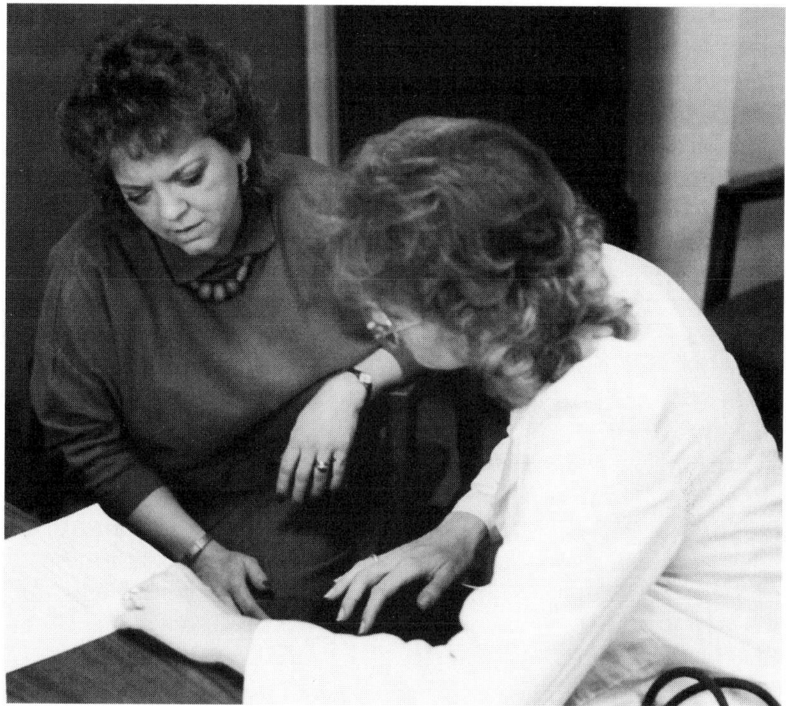

FIG. 25-7 Collaborative position.

Physical barriers send the nonverbal message of protection or *keep your distance*, whether this message is intended or not. When the clinician recognizes barriers, he or she can go around them (such as with an office desk), move them out of the way (such as with charts or crossed arms and legs), or comment on them to soften their effect if they are fixed barriers in the space. It is also important to do *none* of these if it is clear that the barrier is offering the patient or the clinician a sense of protection or safety that is needed at the moment.

Angles of facing are an important component of the interview space. When the clinician and the patient disagree and are sitting directly opposite each other, their physical position can cause them to experience their differences as more of a confrontation than is actually intended. Once the clinician is aware that such a situation exists, he or she can defuse the confrontational aspects by shifting position to change the angle at which he or she is facing the patient. Just a slight angulation off a directly opposite position will begin to ease the tension. If the clinician moves even further into a side-by-side position with the patient, the configuration will more clearly support a collaborative effort between them, in spite of the disagreement (Figure 25-7).

Addressing Mixed Messages

When there is incongruence between verbal and nonverbal modes in the patient's communication, *the nonverbal message more truly reflects the patient's actual feelings and better predicts his or her behavior in response to the issue at hand.* A mixed message means that the patient is not safe enough to tell the clinician how he or she feels. The patient may send a mixed message for a number of reasons: he or she may feel that disagreeing with or questioning the provider may threaten care, feelings may be too unacceptable to acknowledge, or the patient may feel overwhelmed or out of control.

A nonverbal "no" from the patient is signaled by a furrowed brow, slight shaking of the head, a strained voice, breath holding, slightly increased pallor of the face, or tensing of the muscles. The clinician should understand that this "no," even if inconsistent with the patient's verbal response, indicates that the job is not finished. The incongruence must be addressed; if it is not, the patient will not comply with what he or she has agreed to do or will have difficulty or be frustrated in attempting to do it. The physician can also send mixed messages to the patient. If these messages are not acknowledged and discussed, they may send a powerful message about the physician not being trustworthy and will make the encounter feel less safe to the patient.

When dealing with a mixed message from a patient, the physician should try converting an incongruent "no" into a congruent "no" to make it accessible for discussion or to create enough safety for expressing the unexpressed feeling. The two major strategies for doing this are *direct acknowledgment* and *using the language of the third person.*

Direct acknowledgment openly reflects that the physician is receiving two messages from the patient:

> **Physician:** You know, even though you say you'll take the medication, I sense that you have some hesitation about it. If you have some concerns, let's talk about them.

If the patient relaxes or nods in agreement, the physician has succeeded in transforming the incongruent "no" into a congruent "no" that the patient can safely talk about. If the patient withdraws or blanches further, the next strategy may be more useful.

Using the language of the third person avoids direct reflection to the patient. Instead of reflection, this method raises potential questions or fears through linguistic distancing to increase the feeling of safety. The physician can say something such as the following:

> **Physician:** I once worked with a patient in a situation similar to yours who was concerned about starting a new drug.

While saying this, the physician would look carefully at the patient for the nonverbal parameters of agreement such as head nodding, deeper breathing, the return of facial color, or muscular relaxation. If the patient nonverbally agrees and remains silent, the physician can pursue potential concerns further by saying the following:

Physician: This patient had several concerns. One was about possible side effects (watching for nonverbal signs of agreement or disagreement), and another one was the cost (again looking for signs).

By this time, the patient usually feels a clear invitation to explore any of these concerns or to offer additional ones.

APPLICATION TO THE THREE-FUNCTION APPROACH

Each of the nonverbal skills allows the physician to monitor the process of the interaction with the patient in all three functions of the interview. The key is to track the patient's nonverbal output throughout, noticing whether the patient is feeling safe. The following are common strategies for applying the nonverbal skills as the interview progresses.

Function One: Building the Relationship

The nonverbal skills set the form for beginning the relationship with the patient. Well before any words are exchanged, the patient feels the effect of how the interview space is set up. Is the clinician close or distant? Does the physician meet the patient eye-to-eye? Is the desk or chart between them, or is it shared as they work from a side-by-side position?

As the interview begins, the physician should begin matching the patient to join him or her nonverbally in the patient's world. Easy behaviors to match are body lean (left, right, or forward) and volume and rate of speech. If the patient is loud or speaking fast, it is enough for the physician to shift his or her own voice in the direction of more volume and rate without having to match the patient's voice exactly (remember, the patient should not be aware of the matching).

Patients need to know if their provider can tolerate the full expression of their difficulties and suffering. If the physician detects incongruence in the affect the patient is showing versus whether the patient is verbally acknowledging the affect, the physician can use reflection or the language of the third person to help the patient express it more congruently. For example, the physician might say something such as the following:

Physician: Mrs. Jones, you say everything is fine at home with your family, but you seem sad as you speak about them. Is there something else?

Function Two: Assessing the Patient's Problems

The patient who feels safe may give better information. Continuing to monitor nonverbal rapport and nonverbal output of whether the patient feels safe says "I care" in a way that allows the patient to offer spontaneously all the information and associations important to the reason he or she is seeking help. This also makes it easier for the patient to report potentially embarrassing information.

The physician is usually under time pressure and needs to organize the interview to stay on time. Often the physician needs to shift topics, bring closure to a part of the interview, or interrupt a patient who has become tangential in responding to a question. Being in rapport with the patient allows the physician to use the interruption more like a lead and makes it easier for the patient to experience the redirection without closing down on spontaneity or feeling cut off by the physician.

When the physician asks, "Is there anything else?" when developing the agenda at the beginning of the interview and at the end of history taking, he or she should ask this question without delivering a mixed message. Too often the physician accompanies this question by shaking his or her head "no" or pulling away and looking at the chart.

Function Three: Managing the Patient's Problems

The third function of the interview represents a great opportunity for the use of nonverbal skills as the physician works to educate and motivate the patient and develop a treatment plan with him or her. Tension is frequently high between the physician and the patient when they deal with their differences about what is wrong with the patient and what would be helpful to his or her health. Too often the physician feels that the doctor's job is done after the straightforward delivery of diagnostic and treatment information. This simplistic approach can increase the suffering of many patients. Some patients may not understand what the diagnosis means, and others may face major obstacles (e.g., beliefs, emotions, limited financial and personal support, and family commitments) to complying with the physician's recommendations.

Using the nonverbal skills can be extremely important when the physician and patient are working through their differences. Any objection the patient has to the diagnosis or the treatment recommended by the physician may be signaled through the nonverbal channel.

The physician should be in nonverbal rapport with the patient when any diagnosis or treatment is offered. This state of "I am with you" allows the patient to take in the new information more readily and to give it due consideration.

An astute physician can monitor the effect each utterance has on the patient by looking for safe or not-safe responses (many will be subtle). For instance, when the physician offers an explanation of the diagnosis and observes that the patient's body tension has gone up and that the patient is holding his or her breath, the physician should stop and ask what significance (meaning) the explanation seems to have for the patient. The same would apply for any recommendations the physician makes regarding treatment, procedures, or referrals.

Asking whether the patient feels that he or she will be able to adhere to the treatment recommendations is an important part of the interview. If the patient says, "Sure, doc, whatever you say," while turning away and shaking his or her head "no" or if the patient flushes, the physician should know that more work is needed. The physician could move to reflection or to language of the third person to help bring the patient's objection openly to the negotiating table, to figure out a form or plan that might fit better with the patient's concerns and needs, or to offer more information and education.

CONCLUSION

Combining both nonverbal and verbal modes of interaction when working with patients can be tremendously satisfying, because it requires the physician to be more "real" in the professional role in which he or she is encountering patients. Many physicians fear that acknowledging the patient's affect and taking the time to work through the differences in a treatment plan will lead to burnout. The opposite is actually true; the level of honesty and support that is possible when the physician joins the patient more fully in the healing process makes time constraints and the lack of a cure for some presenting problems much easier to bear.

Beginning the nonverbal work slowly and in small segments is useful. The physician should spend time observing nonverbal behavior inside and outside the clinical arena. The physician should focus on one aspect at a time (e.g., shifts in voice tone, flushing or blanching of the face, and which members of a crowd stand in nonverbal synchrony and which do not). It is usually instructive for the physician to notice when he or she moves away or closer to the patient. The physician who takes the time and effort to practice observing nonverbal behaviors will notice that sensory acuity increases steadily and that a new world of discourse and communication opens up.

Additional references are available for further study on each of the aspects of nonverbal behavior.[4,5,6]

REFERENCES

1. Engel G, Schmale A: Conservation-withdrawal: a primary regulatory process for organismic homeostasis. In *Physiology, emotion & psychosomatic illness*, Amsterdam, 1972, Elsevier-Excerpta Medica.

2. Eckman P, Friesen W: *Unmasking the face*, New Jersey, 1975, Prentice-Hall.
3. Maurer, Tindall: Effect of postural congruence on client's perception of counselor empathy, *J Counsel Psychol* 30:158-163, 1983.
4. Carson C: Nonverbal communication in clinical encounters, *Cortland Forum* 129-134, 1990.
5. Milmoe S, Rosenthal R, et al: The doctor's voice: postdictor of successful referral of alcoholic patients, *J Abnormal Psychol* 72:78-84, 1967.
6. Harrigan JA, Rosenthal R: Nonverbal aspects of empathy and rapport in physician-patient interaction. In Blanck et al: *Nonverbal communication in the clinical context*, University Park, Pa, 1986, Penn State University Press.

CHAPTER

26 Use of the Self in Medical Care

Dennis H. Novack

Students and practicing physicians who master the communication skills presented in this text will be more effective clinicians. Yet medicine is also an art. Physicians uniquely combine their knowledge, skills, attitudes, beliefs, and emotional responses to patients in the service of healing. Healing—making patients "whole" again—involves more than curing disease and is promoted by the human connections between physicians and patients. Much of the art of medicine involves physicians using their intuition and personal reactions to patients for their patients' benefit. Self-aware practitioners can be more "skillful artists" in applying their therapeutic interventions.[1]

Personal reactions to patients affect care in many ways. Patients will remind physicians of parents and friends; physicians may like or dislike certain patients based on these impressions. For a variety of reasons they may not fully understand, physicians feel attracted to some patients and repelled by others. Physicians balk at asking certain sensitive questions of any patients. The feelings patients evoke in physicians sometimes aid in understanding a patient's experience in illness and sometimes get in the way. Physicians communicate empathy to some and judge others, nonverbally expressing negative attitudes. They joke freely with some patients and are stiff and formal with others. Physicians may undermine their care of some patients by being too friendly and by trying to do too much, or of other patients by expressing anger with the patients' behavior.

Physicians' personality characteristics, such as obsessiveness, perfectionism, impatience, idealism (or disorganization, patience, and many others), play major roles in their styles of interviewing, the quality and quantity of information they collect, and their abilities in relating to and healing their patients. Since physicians' personal qualities will always affect their behaviors, how can they use self-knowledge in the service of patient care? The answers to this question are related to the physicians' activities in three domains: personal awareness, personal growth, and self-care. This chapter discusses these concepts and illustrates certain points by vignettes from my experiences or from those related by my colleagues in physician support groups.

Physician Personal Awareness

Personal awareness is an essential foundation of practicing the art of medicine. By paying attention to the use of self in patient care, and by discussing a variety of issues with colleagues and friends in formal and informal sessions, students and physicians can continuously enhance their self-awareness. They can make it a practice to notice their feelings in relationship to patients and ask themselves how these feelings are affecting communication. If they hesitate to ask patients certain sensitive questions, they can ask themselves why. If these questions are important to their understanding of a patient's illness, they can find a way to ask such questions in spite of the difficulty (or ask their peers or teachers how they approach these questions). If physicians know that they need to perform a complete examination but want to cut corners, or if they find that they are avoiding interacting with certain patients, they can spend a few minutes reflecting on these feelings and analyzing their origins. For example, trainees in the clinical rotations often indefinitely "defer" breast and genital examinations because of embarrassment and therefore may miss critical findings. Many students feel uncomfortable sitting and talking, or simply listening, to patients who are dying, and they unwittingly cut short their time with these patients or avoid them entirely. This behavior can increase these patients' isolation and pain and rob the students of meaningful interactions.[2] Students can ask themselves what they need to do to overcome feelings and behaviors that may prevent them from offering patients optimal care. The following physician's experience demonstrates how this may be accomplished:

> *Early in my training, I had great difficulty relating to patients around issues of sexuality. I would not ask patients questions about their sex lives or sexual orientation, and I would not examine the breasts of young women patients. I thought it could be sexually stimulating to do so. Confused and ashamed of my feelings, I simply avoided the issues. One day, I admitted a 28-year-old woman with advanced breast cancer to my service. I was horrified to learn that she had a physical examination the year before by a physician who had not done a breast exam.*
>
> *Similarly, I avoided spending time with my dying patients. I was afraid of their pain. I was afraid they would ask me questions I could not answer. I hated feeling helpless and incompetent. I remember one patient who was dying of pancreatic cancer. As he grew more and more jaundiced, I spent less and less time with him, only staying to discuss the most pressing medical issues. One day, I passed his room on rounds and simply waved to him.*

I realized that my avoidance of these difficult and sensitive issues was compromising my medical care. I resolved to overcome my feelings, change my behaviors, talk to trusted colleagues about these issues, and attend conferences and courses that could help me improve my care of patients in these domains.

Students and physicians can also increase self-awareness by reflecting on and discussing with others a variety of topics related to the effects of physicians' personal issues on medical care.[3] It is best for physicians to have these discussions with peers with whom they can be honest and who will be honest in their feedback. Although a full understanding of these issues may develop only over many years, it is worthwhile to begin addressing certain topics from the beginning of medical education. These topics include core beliefs, the effects of family of origin, gender, and culture on one's care of patients, attitudes toward vulnerability and death, love, attraction, and anger in patient care, and medical mistakes.

Students' core beliefs about themselves as future physicians will affect their patient care. If they believe that medicine is a calling, rather than just a job, they are more likely to be tolerant of the stresses of training and to feel more satisfaction with patient care. If they believe that their roles as physicians encompass attention to psychologic and social aspects of illness, they are more likely to explore these issues with their patients. If they have certain "dysfunctional beliefs,"[4] they are likely to experience more stress in training. These dysfunctional beliefs include strong convictions that any limitation in knowledge is a personal failing, that responsibility is to be borne alone by physicians, that altruistic devotion to work and denial of self is desirable, that keeping one's uncertainties and emotions to oneself is professional, and that perfection is an achievable goal.

A student's attitudes, feelings, and behaviors concerning such issues as intimacy, anger, and conflict resolution are often influenced by patterns in the student's family of origin. The student learns first from his or her family about the nature, benefits, and pitfalls of caring, about the roles of the caregiver, about the balance of giving and receiving, about the communicative aspects of illness, and about how to respond to distress. These dynamics are fundamentally important to the physician-patient relationship. Patients may remind physicians of family members with similar problems or behavioral patterns. An unrecognized identification of patients with family members can elicit feelings, including fears of harming the patient, of inadequacy, of loss of control, and of addressing certain difficult topics.[5]

Attitudes about gender roles influence communication with those of the opposite sex. These attitudes, shaped by family and societal norms, can affect patient care and physicians' ability to accept feedback from colleagues of the opposite sex. Similarly, sociocultural norms influence physicians' attitudes toward acceptable illness behaviors, obesity, sexual behaviors, geriatric patients, "family values," the importance of work, and many other emotionally charged issues. Moreover, medical training probably constitutes a distinct culture that facilitates socialization into the profession. The culture of medical training and the culture of the individual hospital can affect physicians' medical care in many ways, and self-awareness can mitigate some of the negative effects. The following personal experience illustrates one way this can happen:

> *The stresses of training and shared misery bound our resident group together, but also fostered an "us against them" mentality toward our patients. We called patients "crocks" and "gomers," and every new admission was a "hit." We spent much more time talking about surgical service "dumps" and the intellectual challenges of certain difficult diagnoses than the suffering and humanity of our patients. One day, a senior resident told me with dismay that she had seen the obituary of one of our "dirtbag" alcoholic patients who had died a few days before. She was shocked to learn that he had been a man of great accomplishment and a real contributor to his community until alcoholism had brought him so low in his last years. She had the sudden realization that our name calling had been a way to avoid connecting certain patients' anxiety and despair with our own. She said to me, with emotion, "My God—something like this could happen to me someday." She vowed to never call a patient a "dirtbag" again.*

Physicians' love and caring for patients contribute to patients' experience of physician empathy and can be healing. However, this love and caring are beneficial only if framed within clear, mutually understood boundaries. Sometimes, perhaps because of unmet personal needs, physicians send unintended messages or become too emotionally invested in certain patients. For physicians in small towns, whose neighbors and friends become patients, and for physicians whose family members fall ill, setting clear boundaries may be especially difficult. Because physician-patient relationships often engender a special intimacy, there is the potential for powerful feelings of attraction to be aroused in both the caregiver and the patient. By understanding their emotional reactions to patients, physicians can set appropriate affective boundaries that allow them to be objective yet connect with patients.[6] The following personal report provides an example:

> *When I was an intern, I remember spending a great deal of time with a young woman diabetic patient who had taken an insulin overdose after an argument with her boyfriend. I offered her empathy and understanding, talked to her about the importance of*

getting counseling, and explored ways that she could improve her social situation and respond more appropriately to stress. The Sunday after her discharge, she paged me and asked if she could see me in the hospital lobby. Though I was having a busy on-call day, I met with her, listened to her latest problems with her boyfriend, and held her hand as she cried. She asked if we could have lunch the next day. I agreed.

I realized that meeting her for lunch was inappropriate, but had felt that doctors needed to be available for their patients and should be able to "go the extra mile" to help them. I had been flattered that she found me so helpful and enjoyed feeling competent in my counseling skills, at a time when my feelings of competence were being otherwise challenged by the sick and dying patients on my service. I probably was also attracted to her, and enjoyed the intimacy of our conversations. I realized, though, that responding to my own needs was undermining my ability to help her. At lunch the next day, I told her of my discomfort and discussed the need for setting appropriate professional boundaries if I were to continue caring for her in the outpatient clinic.

Understanding your attitudes about anger can be helpful in patient care, since illness, suffering, and death often engender angry feelings for patients and their families. Reacting to patients' or their families' anger with anger can be destructive. For physicians to be effective in responding to anger, they need to know the kinds of patients that elicit an angry reaction in them, their own usual responses to their own anger and the anger of others (e.g., do they overreact, placate, blame others, suppress feelings, or become super-reasonable?), and their underlying feelings when they become angry (e.g., feeling rejected, humiliated, or unworthy). Such self-awareness is the starting point for physicians learning to react to anger in a way that contributes to conflict resolution and communicates empathy.

Perhaps no other aspect of medical care demands more attention to self-awareness than the issue of medical mistakes. Being human, all physicians make mistakes. Sometimes these mistakes lead to patient morbidity and death. Physicians who use denial and blame others are not likely to learn from their mistakes. Those who accept responsibility for a mistake and discuss it are more likely to make constructive changes in their practices.[7] To learn from mistakes, physicians must examine the attitudes, feelings, and behaviors that led to the mistake, as demonstrated in the example of the following young attendings' experience:

Preparing for my first rotation as an attending on the inpatient wards, I asked the most popular attending in the hospital if he had any advice. He said, "Well, I'll tell you my secret. Every evening, I go to the pharmacy and look up the orders on all patients admitted to my service. I find out the diagnoses and look up anything I don't know. The next morning, when the team presents the new patients to me, I'm never wrong. They think I'm brilliant!" I was appalled. Students and residents were having a hard enough time struggling to know enough without this attending presenting a false ideal of the all-knowing physician.

Still, the pressures of inpatient medicine can be intense, and most students and house staff had had the experience of feeling embarrassed on rounds that they did not know some piece of information. As an attending, I soon learned the device of turning questions back to the team when asked a question I could not answer. Usually someone on the team knew the answer, and I could add information that I did know about the subject. It seemed a benign form of deception, but I was caught one day, nevertheless.

I was attending on an inpatient service when my resident asked me about a patient we had admitted several days before. This middle-aged man had come to the hospital with a cellulitis and fever and was now improving on IV antibiotics. He had a benign medical history and otherwise normal examination results. The resident told me that one of the patient's blood cultures had come back with a positive result for Enterobacter, *and he asked me if we should alter our antibiotic therapy. I was not sure of the answer, so I hedged. I asked him if the bacteria could have been a contaminant. He replied, "Well, I drew the blood from his groin, so it was a dirty stick. It was the only one of four cultures that was positive, so I guess it could have been." This was an excellent resident who in many respects had more up-to-date knowledge of inpatient medicine than I did, so I assumed he was right. In any case, the patient was improving by all measures, so we agreed that we would keep him on his current regimen. I did not know that* Enterobacter *was rarely a contaminant. Apparently the resident did not know it either but allowed that it was a possibility based on his assumption of my greater experience. Unfortunately, the patient developed a septic condition and died within a week.*

In the end, it turned out that my guess had been correct—subsequent cultures confirmed that his sepsis was due to Escherichia coli, *and the* Enterobacter *had actually been a contaminant. However, it would have been appropriate to start him on broadened antibiotic coverage, which would have been active against* E. coli *as well. The story of his final illness was complicated, and other factors played a role in the outcome. I'll never know if starting a new antibiotic would have saved him. Still, I was left with the knowl-*

edge and sadness that my need to be seen as a bright attending physician could have contributed to his death. I now freely admit my ignorance when asked questions that stump me, and I will not let misplaced feelings of pride affect my medical therapy.

Personal Growth

Attention to personal awareness is essential for personal growth. Attention to activities that promote personal awareness and growth can help physicians develop the maturity and sense of well-being that allow them to focus on patients' problems. Scholars have delineated the components of well-being:

1. *Self-acceptance*—respect and acceptance of one's past life and present identity
2. *Positive relations with others*—includes the ability to have warm, trusting, and intimate relationships
3. *Autonomy*—the ability to act from a stable sense of self and values without needing the approval of others to do what is right
4. *Environmental mastery*—the ability to advance in the world and change it creatively
5. *Sense of purpose in life*—gives one a sense of direction and meaning in work and personal life[8]

A *commitment to personal growth,* that one will continue to develop one's potential, grow and expand as a person, and grow in self-knowledge, helps physicians to develop the sense of well-being essential for optimal patient care.

Medical school can be a challenge to developing a sense of well-being. The press of work tempts students to ignore their relationships with lovers, family, and friends. Some superiors are abusive and some ask students to behave unethically. At times the rigors of clinical work lead students and trainees to feel overwhelmed, anxious, and demoralized. Students must create a context in their medical training for discussions with peers about the stresses of training, personal reactions to patient care, and personal development. Many medical schools have programs to enhance student well-being and personal growth. There are a wide variety of activities, including support, Balint, and literature in medicine discussion groups, that have proved valuable, as well as inclusion of personal reflection activities in behavioral science and clinical skills curricula.[3,9] If a school does not offer such programs, class representatives can work with deans to inaugurate them. Students who begin a pattern of attending to personal awareness, growth, and self-care during their first year of medical school can "immunize" themselves against, or at least prepare for, the stresses to come. Personal awareness and growth can be difficult and sometimes painful for students and physicians, but their rewards often are increased personal freedom and personal and professional satisfaction.

Self-Care

Trainees and physicians cannot be maximally effective in their patient care unless they attend to self-care. Physicians who are unhappy and distracted by personal problems are less available emotionally for their patients and may take a pessimistic view of patients with similar problems. Some students and physicians who are unhappy in their personal relationships use patient care as a way of escape. Patients may be more appreciative than significant others. Patient care has unending potential for commitment, and an adage among house staff is "the longer you stay in the hospital, the longer you stay." Students and physicians who use patient care as an escape often find that their personal conflicts grow worse and that they are putting themselves at risk for burnout and other emotional problems.[10]

Physicians who are very good at prioritizing the tasks in a busy practice typically spend little time prioritizing the tasks needed to have a satisfying personal life. The ability to connect with patients often depends upon physicians' abilities to care for and respect themselves. This process involves active attention to balancing school or work and personal lives, building a support network, joining groups that meet regularly for mutual support, nourishing relationships with significant others, setting aside time for exercise, and actively maintaining some social life and outside interests. Self-care also involves heeding the warning signs of dysfunction. Mental health counselors can often be helpful when relationship problems begin interfering with work. Moreover, physicians have high rates of alcoholism, drug addiction, and depression, all of which can be effectively treated. Physicians who recognize these illnesses early and seek help for them can prevent serious future problems.

In summary, physicians are most effective when they can use their personal reactions to patients for their patients' benefit. Physicians are better able to experience and communicate the empathy that is crucial to patient care when they attend to and develop their abilities to use themselves as instruments of diagnosis and therapy. By focusing on personal awareness, growth, and self-care, they promote their development into physicians who are capable not only of curing disease but of healing illness as well.

REFERENCES

1. Novack DH: Therapeutic aspects of the clinical encounter, *J Gen Intern Med* 2(5):346-355, 1987.

2. Novack DH: Adrienne, *Ann Intern Med* 119(5):424-425, 1993.
3. Novack DH et al: Calibrating the physician: physician personal awareness and effective patient care, *JAMA* 278:502-509, 1997.
4. Martin AR: Stress in residency: a challenge to personal growth, *J Gen Intern Med* 1(4):252-257, 1986.
5. Marshall AA, Smith RC: Physicians' emotional reactions to patients: recognizing and managing countertransference, *Am J Gastroenterol* 90(1):4-8, 1995.
6. Farber ND, Novack DH, O'Brien M: Love, boundaries and the patient-physician relationship, *Arch Intern Med* 157:2291-2294, 1997.
7. Wu AW et al: Do house officers learn from their mistakes? *JAMA* 265(16):2089-2094, 1991.
8. Ryff CD, Singer B: Psychological well-being: meaning, measurement, and implications for psychotherapy research, *Psychother Psychosom* 65:14-23, 1996.
9. Novack DH et al: Personal awareness and professional growth: a proposed curriculum, *Med Encounter* 13(3):2-8, 1997.
10. Vaillant GE, Sobowale NC, McArthur C: Some psychologic vulnerabilities of physicians, *N Engl J Med* 287(8):372-375, 1972.

CHAPTER

27 Using Psychologic Principles in the Medical Interview

When and if patient encounters become difficult or problematic, this text recommends that the interviewer use higher-order interviewing skills to increase the efficiency and effectiveness of the interaction. This chapter focuses on examining the patient's psychology and behavior to provide patient-specific information that will guide the clinician toward more effective higher-order interventions. Numerous psychologic theories and therapies have been applied to the medical setting, many with useful insights. Given the plethora of "schools" of psychology, however, we will focus on the two most influential psychologic models for pragmatic suggestions to improve troubled physician-patient relationships: (1) the psychodynamic model and (2) the cognitive-behavioral model. The interested reader is referred to other sources for information about other psychologic approaches.[1]

The chapter first presents some basic principles of each of the models and then discusses a typical case to which these psychologic principles can be applied.

THE PSYCHODYNAMIC MODEL: BASIC CONCEPTS

Psychic Conflict

One of the key contributions of Freud and subsequent psychodynamic thinkers has been the elaboration of the concept of psychic conflict. This concept asserts that the mind is subjected to internal, generally unconscious conflicts between drives, feelings, or strivings (e.g., aggression, sex, independence, and dependence) and learned fears of the environmental or intrapsychic consequences of these feelings. The particular pattern and expression of basic feelings versus learned fears is infinitely variable from individual to individual.[2,3]

An example of psychic conflict is a great fear of anger. This fear may be innate, or may be developed in the superego from the internalization of parental values. A fear of aggression also may be learned because of childhood experiences of being punished for anger. Furthermore, this fear may be conscious or entirely unconscious. To elaborate on this example, consider a patient who has to wait for 2 hours to see the doctor. He is probably angry. When the doctor finally arrives, the doctor might say something like this:

> **Physician:** I'm sorry to have kept you waiting so long.

Some patients might be willing to express their irritation:

> **Patient:** Your secretary promised me that you wouldn't be running behind today. I've already missed some important appointments.

Patients who are able to acknowledge their irritation (or anger) in this way do not demonstrate evidence of a conflict or fear of anger. However, another patient may become tense and monosyllabic and say, perhaps with a slightly sarcastic tone, something like the following:

> **Patient:** No, Doctor. I know you are very busy. I don't mind waiting. I'm not angry. What good would it do anyway to get angry?

This patient's response demonstrates psychic conflict. Conflict can be conscious to the patient—that is, the patient may be aware of feeling uncomfortable about the admission of angry feelings. He may be aware that he is angry but may be afraid to admit this, thinking the doctor might not take good care of him if he admits he is angry.

Another patient, also consciously aware of angry feelings, may experience conflict because he thinks something like "anger is bad" or "nice people don't get angry." Therefore, when asked about anger, the patient may be aware that he is angry, but because he thinks anger is a "bad" thing to feel, he may deny the feeling when asked about it by the doctor. On the other hand, conflict can be unconscious—that is, the patient may not even be aware that he is feeling angry. Theoretically, the patient's superego or mechanisms of defense operate unconsciously to "protect" the patient from the conscious experience of anger, which would cause the patient to feel uncomfortable or anxious. Thus, when a patient tells the doctor that he is not angry, he may in fact be telling the truth as he believes it. However, the doctor may be aware of the other side of the patient's feelings because of other, perhaps more subtle cues—for example, incongruity between the patient's verbal statements and nonverbal rigidity or profuse or excessive denial.[4]

Understanding the basic principles of psychic conflict is central to good patient management. Many experienced physicians intuitively understand psychic conflict, but more sophisticated understanding can help physicians manage many complex and problematic situations.

Mechanisms of Defense

An understanding of the mechanisms of defense follows logically from an appreciation of psychic conflict. Mechanisms of defense are psychologic maneuvers that operate to protect an individual from anxiety resulting from the expression or conscious awareness of inner drives, needs, or strivings.

In the example described previously, if the individual was unaware of his own anger, it was because of the mechanism of "denial" that operated to protect him from awareness of the anger that would have created internal anxiety.

There are many other mechanisms of defense in addition to denial. Some other defenses are *projection, reaction formation, isolation of affect, conversion,* and *sublimation.*[5] These other defense mechanisms can be illustrated by considering the patient described previously, who has been waiting for 2 hours. *Projection* refers to the mechanism through which the patient's own forbidden feeling or impulse is attributed (or "projected") onto others. For example:

Physician: I'm sorry to have kept you waiting so long.
Patient: I'm not angry, Doctor, but your nurse and I had a disagreement about my blood pressure, and I think she put my file at the bottom of your folders.

Reaction formation refers to the reversal of the forbidden feeling into its opposite. Without ever reaching the level of conscious awareness, the patient may turn his anger into its opposite:

Physician: I'm sorry to have kept you waiting so long.
Patient: That's OK. I'm just grateful you have time for me at all.

Isolation of affect does not deny the presence of the feeling itself but, instead, enables the patient to dissociate himself from the emotions associated with the usual expression of the feeling. For example:

Physician: I'm sorry to have kept you waiting so long.
Patient: It's OK, I guess, but I've gotten very nervous waiting so long. (Patient demonstrates no visible or verbal signs of affective arousal.)

Conversion refers to the displacement of the feeling onto a physical or body part. For example:

Physician: I'm sorry to have kept you waiting so long.
Patient: That's OK, but my stomach pain has been getting worse and worse. I thought you would never come.

Sublimation is a higher-level, more "mature" defense because it effectively turns the energy from conflictual feelings into productive activity. For example:

> **Physician:** I'm sorry I kept you waiting so long.
> **Patient:** It was a long time, but I was able to get some work done.

Physicians who understand the principles of defense mechanisms and can recognize common patterns will be able to provide more psychologically informed care to their patients. Reading can help physicians learn these patterns, but in general the physician needs a specialized learning environment with clinical supervision to master the principles.[6]

Individualized long-term supervision by an expert clinician of the care for specific patients is one way to learn how defense mechanisms operate in longitudinal patient relationships. "Balint" groups, named after the psychiatrist Michael Balint, are another mechanism for the development of such skills. In Balint groups, a group of practicing physicians meets regularly (e.g., every week or every month) with an expert to review complex patients.[7] Finally, clinicians can attend brief (one-day), more extensive (weekly), or more longitudinal training programs (one half day every week) to attain added skills.

Resistance and Management of Resistance

Resistance refers to the tenacity with which patients tend to cling to their defenses. Defenses usually operate unconsciously to protect patients from anxiety. Thus, when a defense is challenged, the patient will usually resist the uncovering of a defense.

For example, a patient has been kept waiting and has already denied that he is angry. The physician may continue to insist that the patient appears angry. If confronted directly, the patient may become even more insistent that he is not angry and say something like the following:

> **Physician:** I'm sorry to have kept you waiting so long.
> **Patient:** I'm not angry, Doctor, but your nurse and I had a disagreement about my blood pressure, and I think she put my file at the bottom of your folders.
> **Physician:** Well, if you think my nurse has interfered with your care, I can certainly understand why you might feel angry about that.
> **Patient:** I told you I am <u>not</u> angry!

In general, physicians need to respect a patient's resistance and not challenge it unless the mechanism of defense leads the patient to maladaptive behavior. To give an example: the patient who has denied his anger may be so tense, so irritable, and so uncooperative that the physician finds working with him difficult.

The management of resistance usually involves some attempt to draw attention to the resistance to facilitate the expression of the underlying feeling. The technical words used to describe these interventions are *confrontation* and *interpretation*. Some physicians intuitively use confrontation and interpretation quite effectively, but attaining a high degree of skill in the management of resistance usually requires dedicated and systematic study with clinical supervision.

Confrontation is an unfortunate choice of words because it implies some degree of conflict between the caregiver and the patient. In fact, the skillful use of confrontation describes the attempt to bring an emotional issue to the awareness of the patient in such a way as to cause as little embarrassment as possible and in a manner that can maximize the chances of the patient being able to accept the awareness of the emotion. Acceptance, gentleness, thoughtfulness, and the willingness to be wrong are all characteristics that can help a physician confront a patient with maladaptive resistance. In the case described previously, the physician might comment as follows:

Physician: OK, I guess I was wrong about saying you might be angry. All I meant to say was that I could understand how you might feel a little bothered if you think my nurse had manipulated my files to keep you waiting so long.

Patient: Well, of course I feel bothered. Wouldn't you be?

Physician: I can't be exactly sure how I would feel, but the important thing now is how I can be of help to you.

Interpretation refers to the uncovering of the basic conflict itself. For example, the physician who knows this patient well might try to help him understand and "work through" this conflict about anger. This is the core process in psychodynamic psychotherapy[8] and is generally not a part of the practice of most general physicians. Nevertheless, many physicians are successful in offering patients intuitive interpretations that help them attain genuine insight or growth. However, interpretation in the service of insight and subsequent working through of psychic conflicts are generally best left to formal psychotherapy or only attempted with close supervision.

Support

At first glance the concept of "support" appears simple. Examined more deeply, however, being supportive to patients can become quite complex. Trying to be "nice," "sensitive," or "warm" is part of good medical care and as such is straightforward.

When patients demonstrate resistance, however, or act in any maladaptive manner, the question of support becomes more problematic. In the patient who manifests a clear defense against anxiety or resistance, a supportive intervention becomes one that, technically, supports the patient's defense. For example, if the patient insists that he is not angry, the doctor supports this defense by making a comment such as:

Physician: OK, I guess I was wrong about what I thought was anger on your part.

Werman[9] has written an important book describing the complexity of supportive interventions. According to Werman, support may be difficult because the physician can be most supportive only when he or she understands the prominent defenses of the patient. Thus it is not always in the patient's best interest for the physician to support defenses. For example, the patient who denies serious illness may not take medications regularly. Similarly, the patient with hypertension may say, "I feel too healthy to have a stroke." The physician who supports such a patient will make the patient feel less anxious in the short run, but at the cost of life-threatening and maladaptive behavior on the patient's part. Confrontation or interpretation, on the other hand, increases patient anxiety in the short run but may lead to more adaptive behavior in the long run.

Thus the decision to emphasize support, which may decrease anxiety in the short run, or to emphasize confrontation and interpretation, which generally increases anxiety, can be difficult. Inappropriate support may at times be dangerous or reinforce maladaptive behavior. On the other hand, the effort to confront patients' defenses generally produces anxiety for the patient and usually for the physician as well. Therefore clear-headed understanding of the difference between support and uncovering can help physicians learn to appreciate these important differences and make better decisions about intervention.

Transference

The concept of *transference* refers to the tendency of patients to displace onto the physician feelings that appropriately belong to other important people.[11] This is a phenomenon that occurs in all relationships but becomes pronounced in doctor-patient relationships because the physician often becomes such an important person with accompanying symbolic power to the patient.

For purposes of illustration, consider again the patient who has been kept waiting for 2 hours to see the doctor. Perhaps this is a patient who feels slighted by many of the important people in his life: his father always kept him waiting and his wife does the same. It is quite likely that the patient will be especially hurt and angry at the physician who keeps him waiting because he "transfers" the anger and hurt from his personal life to the physician who acts in similar ways or who acts in ways to provoke these painful memories. The physician may be the unwitting victim of these "surplus" emotions.

At times, physicians may be told directly about transference feelings. A patient might say something like this:

> **Patient:** You're just like everyone else. Everything else is more important than I am. My father always kept me waiting. My wife does the same. I'm used to it, Doctor. Don't worry.

More commonly, the patient is unaware of transference feelings. The patient assumes these feelings are entirely normal (they are what he or she is used to), and the patient is unaware that the feelings gain a special charge because of his or her emotional history. However, the physician who understands transference will appreciate these problems when noticing the presence of the patient's "surplus" feelings that do not seem appropriate to the clinical situation.

Just being aware of the phenomenon of transference can help physicians cope with difficult situations. However, using this understanding in work with patients can be complex, and physicians interested in making these skills a part of their routine practice generally find the need to obtain further training.

Countertransference

Countertransference refers to the feelings caregivers develop in response to patients. These feelings emanate from the caregiver's personal life experiences. Just as patients have transference feelings to doctors, physicians experience countertransference to patients. At times, patients remind physicians of important people in their own lives. For example, an irritable geriatric patient may remind a physician of his or her own troubled relationship with a parent, or a nonadherent adolescent may provoke feelings similar to the feelings a physician has toward his or her own child.

The physician's care of patients may become compromised or unreasonably emotional because of these countertransference feelings. This happens frequently in the routine practice of medicine. It is unavoidable. However, the physician who is aware of the principles of countertransference may realize the inappropriateness of his or her feelings and gain better emotional control for the benefit of the physician and the patient as well.[11]

Physicians may have feelings toward patients that are not just countertransference. Dying patients may provoke sympathy, sadness, or fear, and angry patients may induce anger, or frustration, among other feelings. Personal awareness and acceptance of feelings toward patients help the physician cope with the patient and with his or her own attitudes toward practicing medicine (see Chapter 26, "Use of the Self in Medical Care").

COGNITIVE-BEHAVIORAL MODEL: BASIC CONCEPTS

Primacy of Cognition

The cognitive-behavioral model of psychologic functioning emphasizes the profound impact of cognitive processes on subsequent behavior and feelings. According to this theory, what we think about something (even though we may not be aware of the thought at the time) determines what we feel about it and what we do. Developed by Aaron Beck and others,[12] this approach examines the effect of deeply ingrained maladaptive or dysfunctional thought processes on a patient's overall functioning. With this approach in mind, cognitive-behavioral interventions focus on interrupting and changing these dysfunctional thought patterns.

According to cognitive models (as is the case with psychodynamic models), our early experiences are powerful in shaping our future reactions. The cognitive view is that in our early years we acquire a set of "core assumptions" or "schemas" about the meaning of experiences and that these assumptions shape the way we think about events for the rest of our lives. These core assumptions influence our initial thought when an event occurs and in turn influence our feelings and behaviors. The first thought is often rapid, automatic, and transient and may at first be difficult to identify. Beck and others have identified several common categories of dysfunctional automatic thoughts that can lead to inappropriate feelings and behaviors. Arbitrary inference (described below) is one such category that has the potential to lead to significant subsequent dysfunction.

Arbitrary Inference

Arbitrary inference refers to patterns of automatic, but mistaken, conclusions patients make based on certain types of environmental input.

To exemplify the process of arbitrary inference, consider again the patient whom the doctor kept waiting for 2 hours. Imagine more background information on this patient: he was the oldest of a family of five and felt (bitterly) that his parents devoted most of their time and attention to his younger siblings. This left him automatically thinking, "I am less important than the others," whenever someone in authority paid less attention to him than he thought he deserved. In response to the physician's apology for being late, this patient might say resentfully:

Patient: That's OK, doctor. I'm used to waiting for others.

The physician who recognizes this maladaptive pattern of thinking may be able help the patient "reality-test" by pointing out something such as the following:

Physician: I realize the fact that I kept you waiting may feel like I have done something personal to you. Please be reassured that the unexpected emergency I had to attend to was unavoidable, and that everyone else in the office has also been kept waiting. You now have my undivided attention.

Operant Conditioning

The contribution of behavioral principles to cognitive-behavioral psychology lies in understanding the importance of stimuli from the environment in shaping subsequent behavior. Operant conditioning theory focuses on understanding the origins of behavior (and feelings) through understanding the contingencies (reinforcement and punishment) that follow predictably from certain behaviors.[13,14] According to this view, behavior and related affects can be changed by consistently changing these contingencies. Reinforcement of desired behaviors is considerably more effective in producing lasting behavior change than punishment of undesirable behaviors.

Consider the angry patient who has been kept waiting. Perhaps he has been physically punished in early life for expressing any anger. Thus he has "learned" never to express anger. In response to the physician's statement about being late, the patient might respond in a sullen manner, with a remark such as the following:

Patient: That's OK, doctor, I know you are very busy.

The physician who can recognize this unexpressed anger can often facilitate rapport by changing the contingency—accepting, and not punishing, the expression of irritation:

Physician: I appreciate your understanding. However, many people do feel irritated when their doctors keep them waiting. So, again, I am sorry to have kept you waiting and will now listen carefully to your problems.

GEORGE: A CASE STUDY INTEGRATING PSYCHODYNAMIC AND COGNITIVE-BEHAVIORAL INTERVENTIONS

Can the primary care physician attain sufficient understanding of psychodynamic and cognitive-behavioral approaches to apply them usefully in clinical practice? While these approaches represent complex theoretical systems that require years of focused study and practice to master, the central principles elaborated above can be used by most physicians. Of course, physicians interested in developing more proficient skills in this domain will need to dedicate time and effort to study, practice, and receive feedback from peers or experts.

The common problem of lower back pain, described in the following example, illustrates ways in which the busy physician may begin to apply both psychodynamic and cognitive-behavioral insights to improve the quality and outcome of the clinical encounter.

The medical history is presented from the patient's point of view:

> *I am a 52-year-old, highly skilled automobile mechanic. I have been a good husband, father, and provider for my wife and children for 30 years. I am seeing Dr. Smith about lower back pain. It started several years ago from lifting at work and now is much worse. I haven't been able to work for several weeks and haven't been much use at home either. I don't like being useless and dependent on my wife.*
>
> *I was very pleased with Dr. Smith at first. He diagnosed my problem as "back strain" and said I would get better soon. He put me on analgesics and bed rest and told me to lose 30 pounds.*
>
> *Unfortunately, my pain grew progressively worse and I was less and less pleased with Dr. Smith and each appointment that followed. The CT scan did not show "anything" to explain the pain, and I insisted on an MRI. Dr. Smith reluctantly agreed to the MRI and seemed to say, "I told you so" when the MRI failed to show any other significant problem.*
>
> *I started to get the impression that the whole thing was being blamed on me and my weight. Each time the back got worse I had to push for an urgent appointment for stronger pain medication. I got the impression that Dr. Smith wasn't happy about all this and was starting to see me as a burden and a failure. I was already pretty fed up about the back trouble, and his attitude made me feel worse.*
>
> *Then Dr. Smith started asking questions about my personal life and my sleep pattern and whether I was depressed. I said that I was no more depressed than anyone else would be in the circumstances. He finally said that I was suffering from "clinical depression."*
>
> *Now it was clear to me that he saw me as a mental case and thought my back pain was all in my head. I didn't like what he said, but I didn't get angry. I just said that I wanted to see a back expert because I no longer trusted his opinion. I walked out and never returned.*

So what went wrong? There are no bad guys in this common story. George's physician was probably polite, conscientious, and sensible, as well as aware of relevant psychiatric and physical diagnoses. George himself represents a common type of patient. As the patient continued to suffer, the relationship deteriorated into an unsatisfactory one for patient and for physician. The core psychodynamic and cognitive-behavioral principles delineated above can provide guidance regarding the use of higher-order but pragmatic interventions for general medical practice.

Psychodynamic Understanding and Interventions

Psychodynamic principles suggest that conflicts about anger and dependency lead to significant psychic anxiety. Regardless of the extent of objective findings to explain his back pain, George's subjective pain and dysfunction understandably led to psychic conflict and the use of defense mechanisms and resistance to deal with the conflicts.

Being out of work and dependent led to feelings of anxiety and low self-esteem. George was angry about his situation and about the physician's inability to help. Rather than express his anger or gracefully accept his dependency, George felt more anxiety, which probably exacerbated his back pain. He used the defense of denial ("I didn't get angry, I just walked out") to help him deal with the anxiety. George also probably had some element of conversion (somatization) to help him cope with the stress of back pain, dependency, anger, and whatever other stresses were ongoing in his life.

George's comments about the physician's view of him as a burden and a failure probably reflected some elements of transference to previously important authority figures in his life (perhaps his father?) who disapproved of him if he did not perform "adequately." Furthermore, if Dr. Smith was indeed annoyed, Dr. Smith, himself, may have had some countertransference feelings about dependent individuals reaping undeserved benefits (of unemployment or analgesics).

What could the psychodynamically informed physician do to improve the problem encounter? From a dynamic point of view, interventions that technically were considered supportive were not working with this patient. Interventions that recognized, accepted, and supported the pain led to increased pain, increased analgesic use, and increased dependency.

Psychodynamically, the most important first principle here is to address the emotional distress and empathize with the patient's predicament. Direct questions from the patient about the underlying cause, the pain, and further medical tests should be temporarily postponed until after the physician addresses the patient's emotional turmoil.

By the time the patient starts to exit the relationship, it may be too late for psychodynamically informed interventions. However, appropriate interventions to help prevent rupture of the relationship would start with basic rapport-building skills (reflection, legitimation, partnership, support and respect) and then address the defenses and the underlying emotional turmoil and conflicts:

Patient: Doc, I'm not getting anywhere with you on this. I'm leaving. I need a specialist.

Physician: Mr. Jones, I will be happy to work with you (partnership) regarding a referral if that is what you want. Before you walk out, I want to make sure you know that I understand how frustrating this has been for you. (reflection)
Many people would feel the same way. (legitimation)
If you want to stay a few more moments, I will do what I can to help you with this and work with you to develop a plan. (support and partnership)
I also want you to know that I am impressed by how well you are coping with a terribly difficult situation—you are in great pain, out of work, and feeling lousy—and without any real answers as yet. (respect)
I realize it must be terribly hard for you to feel so dependent on others. I am sure it also makes you angry. (interpretation of conflicts about dependency and anger)

Most patients respond positively to this type of empathic intervention. Patients often then begin talking about their conflicts and feelings. If the physician can listen empathically, sufficient rapport may develop to construct a mutually acceptable management plan.

Cognitive-Behavioral Understanding and Interventions

Cognitive-behavioral understandings and interventions most productively coincide with and supplement psychodynamic ones. George demonstrates multiple examples of dysfunctional cognitions with faulty arbitrary inferences. He probably believes the following:

- If I don't support my family, I am not a man.
- If I am not a man, I am not worthwhile.
- Only weak people get depressed.
- If the doctor thinks I am depressed, he must think I am weak.

The physician who understands these arbitrary inferences and their effect on George can make effective interventions to strengthen the doctor-patient relationship and improve George's coping mechanisms. For example:

Physician: I realize it is very upsetting to be out of work. I am sure it makes you feel bad. However, it really takes a lot of strength and courage to cope with being sick. Only the strongest of men are able to handle this kind of disability. I am sure your wife and children accept your temporary disability. I truly believe you will be back to work in a short period of time.

With respect to your thoughts about depression, you are quite right that most people in this situation get very distressed. It is not a sign of weakness. It is very understandable. However, if you let me treat your depression in addition to your back pain, I think I can help you return to better functioning faster.

Cognitive-behavioral psychology also suggests using operant conditioning models to help shape behavior. The most effective contingencies for altering behavior involve rewards for desirable behavior, rather than punishments for undesirable behavior. The physician should understand how to use praise from himself or herself as a source of positive reinforcement for the patient. Small, reachable goals should be established, and considerable praise should be given when these goals are met. The physician should allow the patient to set the goals. For example:

Physician: Mr. Jones, please give me an idea about how much pain medicine you are willing to stick to this week.

or

How much exercise are you willing to commit to?

or

What type of diet are you willing to follow this week?

If the patient and the physician together can develop some mutually agreed-upon goals that are realistic for this patient at this time, the physician's praise for achievement of the goals will reinforce the desired behavior. Reinforcement from other sources, such as the family and the employer, is also useful in difficult situations.

CONCLUSION

This chapter reviews ways for physicians to use the contributions of psychodynamic and cognitive-behavioral psychology to achieve more efficient and effective communication in difficult patient encounters. While these concepts are complex and require considerable training and expertise to master thoroughly, some of the core concepts can be usefully applied by interested clinicians in the routine practice of medical care.

REFERENCES

1. Novack DH: Therapeutic aspects of the clinical encounter, *J Gen Intern Med* 2:347-354, 1987.

2. Cooper AM, Frances AJ, Sack M: The psychodynamic model. In Cavenar JO Jr, editor: *Psychiatry*, vol 1, Philadelphia, 1989, JB Lippincott.
3. Hine FR: *Introduction to Psychodynamics: a conflict-adaptational approach*, Durham, N.C., 1971, Duke University Press.
4. Hall JA: Affective and nonverbal aspects of the medical visit. In Lipkin M Jr, Putnam S, Lazare A, editors: *The medical interview: clinical care, education, and research*, New York, 1995, Springer-Verlag.
5. Freud A: The ego and the mechanisms of defense. In Freud A, editor: *The notes of the writings of Anna Freud*, vol 2, New York, 1966, International Universities Press.
6. Levy ST: *Principles of interpretation*, New York, 1984, Jason Aronson.
7. Balint M: *The doctor, his patient, and the illness*, New York, 1976, International Universities Press.
8. Brenner C: *An elementary textbook of psychoanalysis*, New York, 1955, International Universities Press.
9. Werman D: *The practice of supportive psychotherapy*, New York, 1984, Brunner/Mazel.
10. Nemiah J: *Foundations of Psychopathology*, New York, 1961, Oxford University Press.
11. Smith R: Use and management of physician's feelings during the interview. In Lipkin M Jr, Putnam S, Lazare A, editors: *The medical interview: clinical care, education, and research*, New York, 1995, Springer-Verlag.
12. Beck AT, Haaga DA: The future of cognitive therapy, *Psychotherapy* 29:34, 1992.
13. Dorsett PG: Behavioral and social learning psychology. In Stoudemire A, editor: *Human behavior: an introduction for medical students*, Philadelphia, 1998, JB Lippincott.
14. Skinner BF: *About Behaviorism*, New York, 1974, Vintage Books.

CHAPTER

28 Integrating Structure and Function

This text focuses on the three basic functions of the medical interview with concrete, pragmatic suggestions for physicians to improve the efficiency and effectiveness of their communication with patients. However, the doctor-patient encounter is an extraordinarily subtle, rich, and complex phenomenon, about which even the most experienced physicians and most knowledgeable researchers continue to seek further growth. Thus, while mastery of the basic skills presented in this text yields clear competence, attainment of true clinical excellence requires supplementation of the basic skills with a wide variety of higher-order processes and related skills.

For the purposes of this book, both basic and higher-order skills are implemented using concrete, observable behaviors. Basic skills are relatively straightforward. In fact, most of this book has been devoted to the presentation and illustration of operational definitions of these behaviorally grounded skills.

Higher-order skills reflect more complex behaviors that do not lend themselves so readily to operational definitions. Furthermore, higher-order skills reflect behaviors emanating from complex internal processes that may be even more difficult to describe than the skills themselves. One reason these internal processes remain so undefined is that they often operate unconsciously or only within the partial awareness of the clinician. At times it may be difficult to separate these internal processes from their corresponding outward behavior and skills.

Much of the knowledge of the higher-order skills remains "tacit" or "personal," as described by the philosopher of science Michael Polanyi.[1] As such, they are considerably more difficult to teach and learn than the basic skills. On the other hand, just because these skills are tacit and difficult to teach and learn, physicians should not relegate them to the domain of the intuitive and unteachable.

The task of making the tacit explicit and setting forth the principles of higher-order functioning is well worth the effort. When learners can understand and articulate these principles, they can begin to use them as templates to become more effective self-observers and communicators.

This concluding chapter addresses the most complex, subtle, and important, yet least understood, of the higher-order skills: the ability to integrate structure and function in the medical interview.

The skillful physician operates at all times within an overlapping matrix of structural and functional objectives. Regardless of whatever element of data (structure) the physician may be concerned with obtaining at any one moment of the interview, he or she simultaneously must also attend and respond appropriately to relevant input regarding the emotional and management domains (functions) of the interview process. For example, a question about cardiac history in the family may induce anxiety about a parent's heart attack or a question about exercise. Conversely, when offering an educational message about smoking, the physician may encounter new information concerning cardiac symptoms about which he had been unaware or new anxieties over sexuality.

This chapter describes several processes and principles that can aid physicians in accomplishing integrative goals efficiently and effectively. Understanding and using these processes and principles can help physicians achieve proficiency in integrative communication.

HIGHER-ORDER PROCESSES AND SKILLS

Clinical Reasoning

The study of medical expertise and of the data-gathering approaches of experienced physicians indicates that expert interviews do not necessarily proceed in a completely open-ended manner of unbiased data gathering. That is, the expert medical interviewer does not act as a "blank slate," collecting neutral data for the subsequent development of diagnostic possibilities. From the first moments of meeting patients, experts generate hypotheses and explanatory models. As described by Elstein and colleagues,[2] Kassirer and Gorry,[3] and Kaplan,[4] expert clinicians search for meaning in the patient's diverse complaints by comparing the patient's story with their own cognitive (internal) templates of known illness patterns. This search for meaning by the physician is paralleled by the patient's own search for a satisfactory explanatory model for his or her problem(s).[5]

The search for patterns leads the expert clinician to generate a limited number of explanatory hypotheses, perhaps four or five at most, very early in the interview process. This hypothesis generation reflects the highest degree of clinical expertise and has become the subject of considerable research.[6] At present, however, little is known about the exact nature of this process, and even less is known about how to teach it. After generating diagnostic hypotheses, the expert clinician pursues these possibilities by systematic questioning to test and refine hypotheses and generate new hypotheses, if necessary.

Expertise in clinical reasoning (hypothesis generation and testing) and related processes of decision analysis (to help guide physicians' choices in interviewing and investigation) are important in the efficient and effective practice of clinical medicine. Physicians' understanding and mastery of these principles will become even more important as the practice of medicine becomes increasingly complex. Nurcombe and Gallagher[7] describe a model of medical student education in clinical reasoning that could be an example for other programs.

The mastery of clinical reasoning can be added to the basic skills described in this text. Clinical reasoning enriches basic skills—it does not supplant them. Basic data-gathering skills such as open-ended questions, facilitation, and checking remain just as important within more sophisticated models of interviewing. Furthermore, the importance of the basic skills for rapport development and for education and motivation does not change within a more sophisticated approach.

Clinical Inference and Flexibility

Of all the skills addressed in this text, clinical inference and flexibility are the two most important. Clinical inference refers to the ability to observe the patient and infer what he or she is experiencing (e.g., thoughts, feelings, and concerns). There is limited information on how this clinical intuition can be learned or taught. Understanding nonverbal cues is one element of intuition, but other factors are also important. Clinical experience is invaluable for developing inferential abilities, and imitation from observing experienced physicians at work is also critical.[6]

Flexibility, the other skill of central importance to skilled interviewing, is related to clinical intuition. Flexibility in interviewing is the ability to observe the impact of interventions on patients and respond appropriately and flexibly. The most important rule of flexible interviewing is to "use what works." Since every patient is somewhat different from every other patient, the skilled interviewer must be prepared to change and adapt interventions according to the needs and responses of patients. The better the observational and inferential abilities of the physician, the faster he or she will be able to decide how interventions are working and the more flexible he or she will be in altering behavior to meet the needs and responses of the patient. Flexibility can be considered under several headings: flexibility of language, of style, of agenda, of control, of advice, and of function.

Flexibility of language concerns the physician's efforts to use language and concepts that are readily understood by the patient. Most doctors try to do this, but even so they often either slip into professional jargon or oversimplify, which can cause patients to feel patronized. If in doubt, the physician can ask the patient directly for his or her view about the complexity of the language being used.

Flexibility of style is closely related to flexibility of language. It concerns the physician's efforts to emphasize aspects of his or her personality to which the patient is most responsive. This differential responsiveness is related to transference. Some patients respond best to a doctor who is parental; others need a doctor who comes across more like a friend or peer; others, often but not always older patients, are more cooperative if the doctor's style reminds them of a helpful son or daughter. Skilled physicians adapt themselves to these roles to some degree while not compromising their basic integrity or indulging in phony games.

Flexibility of agenda concerns the physician's adaptation of his or her agenda to fit with the patient's agenda. The highly skilled physician takes care to identify the underlying concerns and expectations that prompted the patient's visit. For reasons that may be unconscious, these true concerns are often not made clear. If underlying concerns are not identified and responded to, the patient may be dissatisfied and subsequently "uncooperative." In effect, the doctor's time will have been wasted.

Flexibility of control concerns the physician's willingness to allow the patient to dictate the process and content of the interaction to varying degrees. Some patients have a strong need to feel in control and will be forthcoming and cooperative only if this need is met.

Flexibility of advice concerns the physician's efforts to modify his or her medical advice in the light of the patient's health beliefs and health habits. Textbook advice may strike some patients as unrealistic or downright bad, in which case they will be dissatisfied and difficult. The doctor again would be wasting time.

Flexibility of function indicates the willingness and ability of the physician to shift among the three functions of the interview, depending on the patient's needs at the moment. While the physician gathers data, the patient's emotional state may demand attention, or similar emotional needs may emerge when the physician discusses a treatment plan. Skillful interviewing requires movement from one function to another as deemed appropriate.

Most of the higher-order processes and skills described in this chapter can be recognized in the expert clinician more easily than they can be described or taught. In general, complex skills can be most easily attained through clinical experience, observation of experts, self-reflection, and supervision.

SIX PRINCIPLES OF INTEGRATIVE, HIGHER-ORDER FUNCTIONING

Observe Your Patient

"Observe your patient" is the cardinal rule of higher-order interviewing. The skilled observer can discriminate enormous and often key diagnostic and management information concerning physical as well as emotional functioning from simple observation of such things as posture, gait, position of the eyes, head, tremor, and clammy skin. Close observation also allows the interviewer to gauge the impact of his or her questions and comments on the patient and "correct" any interventions that have had unintended or negative effects on the patient.

Unfortunately, "Observe your patient" is one of the most commonly violated rules. Without observing the patient closely, nonverbal signals of great importance can easily go unnoticed. Physicians who read the chart while they talk to patients often miss important clues, which can be time saving and crucial for effective diagnosis. To give one example, a very experienced and caring neurologist with whom I worked closely once interviewed a man with Parkinson's disease who started crying when the physician asked a question about his spouse. Although I was able to observe this, the physician missed this dramatic moment entirely because he was reviewing the chart at that moment.

Observe Yourself

The skilled interviewer also pays attention to his or her own emotional reactions. For example, a feeling of frustration, anger, sadness, anxiety, boredom, or the like should be viewed as an opportunity to enrich understanding of the patient and the current doctor-patient relationship. This enriched understanding of the relationship should be viewed as a vehicle for improved efficiency and effectiveness in the encounter, rather than as an obstacle to care.

Just as diagnostic hypotheses are continually generated by the data from the patients' narrative history, physicians should produce relationship hypotheses as they become aware of their own feelings in the interview. For example, physicians who notice that they feel irritated should ask themselves questions about the origin of this frustration:

1. "Why am I irritated now?"
2. "Is it just that I am tired and busy?"
3. "Is there something else about this patient that bothers me?"
4. "Is the patient responding to me like someone else I know who irritates me?" (counter-transference)
5. "Do I remind the patient of someone important in the patient's life that can account for this tension in the relationship?" (transference)

Answers, or hypotheses about answers, lead the skilled interviewer to an altered line of interventions (assessment, management, or rapport development) that results in more efficient and effective interviewing. Interviews that become more efficient and effective involve less of the physician's emotional effort.

When in Doubt, Check

"Checking" has already been described as one of the most important basic skills of assessment (of data) and of management (understanding diagnosis and treatment). It also has special importance as a higher-order, integrative skill. When a physician notices that something is not flowing smoothly in the interview process but does not fully understand the source of the difficulty, the physician should turn to the patient for help in understanding the problem and seeking the resolution. For example:

> **Physician:** It seems to me, Mrs. Jones, that we're getting a little stuck on this issue of the diabetes medication. We seem to be going around in a bit of a circle. Let me repeat to you what I have heard you say so far, and then you can fill in the details.

By reviewing the circumstances of the conversation, the physician allows the patient the opportunity to clarify the source of the problem. Furthermore, while reviewing the interaction sequence, the physician gains the time and perspective to increase his or her understanding of the difficulty and develop new strategies for interventions.

When the Patient Demonstrates an Emotion, Respond to It

Although a skillful interviewer begins all interviews by building rapport, the patient, especially one with acute or chronic illness, usually experiences emotions throughout the interview. If the patient shows anxiety, anger, or sadness, for example, it is almost always best to respond to this emotion immediately. Many interviewers are afraid that they will lose time in the interview or open Pandora's box if they attend to the patient's emotions every time these feelings emerge.

> ***Immediate attention to the emotional domain saves time, certainly in the long run and almost always in the short term. Emotions that are not addressed will be suppressed, only to reemerge in more distressing form later.***

This rule of good interviewing is discussed earlier in the book, regarding rapport development as a basic skill. It is repeated here because of its importance as a higher-order, integrative skill. Most of the difficulty that interviewers encounter with their patients can be addressed by improved attention to the emotional domain of the interview.

Focusing attention on the physician-patient relationship during the interview is a higher-order, integrative skill because it often necessitates (especially for problem patients) the flexible use of the three functions simultaneously or in rapid succession. For example, if the physician notes that the patient seems angry about a recommendation to lose weight, the physician should respond to the anger with a comment like, "It seems that my recommendations to lose weight have made you short tempered with me." The patient's response to the physician's empathic (function one—reflection) comment will contain important information (function two—assessment), which the physician will need to evaluate in order to continue with function three (function three—management) effectively.

Don't Answer Every Question Immediately

Answering questions too quickly is a common mistake that physicians, even experienced and skillful ones, make in their everyday practices. Many questions that patients ask their physicians convey significant emotional distress. If the associated emotional distress is not addressed, the answer may not satisfy the patient, not because the answer is incorrect, but because the answer did not deal with the underlying emotional concern. For example, the patient who has been waiting too long might ask the question (with an irritated tone):

> **Patient:** Doctor, I guess you've been pretty busy today?

The doctor who answers the question without addressing the emotional concern (or loss of rapport) might say something like:

> **Physician:** Yes, I had some unexpected emergencies to deal with.

This reply misses the point of the patient's frustration.

When patients ask questions that emanate from emotional distress, it is usually better to address the emotional distress first or include the response to the emotion in the answer. A better response to the patient's question about the physician's schedule might acknowledge the patient's frustration and offer an appropriate apology. For example:

> **Physician:** I understand your impatience and frustration. I am very sorry. I had several unexpected emergencies about which I had no choice. You now have my undivided attention.

As another example, consider a patient with unexplained abdominal pain, who asks the physician (in an anxious tone), "Doctor, what do you think is wrong with me?" The physician might be tempted to answer the question by saying something like, "Well, it could be a number of things, like irritable colon, diverticulitis, a virus, (and so on)." If the patient is afraid that he might have a cancer like his father, these answers might not be reassuring. A better response would be one that addresses the observed anxiety, for example:

> **Physician:** You seem quite concerned about what might be causing this problem. Can you tell me what diagnosis most worries you?

Alternatively, rapport-building interventions like support and partnership are often effective first responses to questions containing emotional distress. Another response to the question about abdominal discomfort might be the following:

> **Physician:** I will answer your question in a moment. However, before I review the diagnostic possibilities with you, I want to make it clear that I see that you are worried. I want you to know that I do not see any specific possibility of anything serious that should worry you.

Of course, this statement can be made truthfully only if the physician believes there is no serious problem.

In the event that the physician is indeed worried about a potentially serious problem, the physician should still respond to the emotion with support and partnership, as part of (or even before) answering the question. For example:

> **Physician:** I can see that you are worried about the possible meaning of these symptoms. I want you to know that I am going to get an answer for us just as soon as possible and that whatever we find, I will work with you to develop an appropriate management plan. These are the possibilities as I see them . . .

Understand That Patients Are Usually Forgiving of "Mistakes" in the Interview

What about physicians who violate the rules of basic or higher-order interviewing that are described in this text? What effect does this have on their patients?

Physicians often interrupt their patients, overlook key diagnostic cues, miss important emotional messages, and deliver ambiguous management suggestions. Fortunately, for many reasons, patients are generally quite forgiving of their physicians and these "mistakes".

Understanding the forgiving tendency of patients can be helpful to beginning as well as experienced clinicians who are developing or using higher-order, integrative skills. If physicians actually care about their patients and try to help, as most physicians do, this caring comes through to their patients who generally tolerate most interviewing mistakes. The skilled physician who continually observes the patient and himself or herself will have multiple opportunities to rectify these errors. For example, consider the physician who fails to notice or respond to a patient's fear of cancer. The verbal or nonverbal expression of the fear will appear again, giving the physician a second chance to respond appropriately.

The tendency of unacknowledged emotions to recur underscores the importance of addressing emotional or rapport problems as soon as they appear. Despite the fear of opening the gates to a flood of emotions, early attention to emotional distress saves time. Patients are far less forgiving of the physicians whom they feel are "too busy" to care. These are the physicians, in fact, who get sued. "Not caring" is the reason most patients give for starting lawsuits against physicians.[8] It does not take a long time to demonstrate caring to most patients. Most physicians do care about most patients and demonstrate this caring intuitively without recourse to basic or higher-order interviewing skills. The rules and techniques of good interviewing have the greatest applicability to encounters with difficult patients, which presents a problem to the physician perhaps only 5% to 10% of the time.

Integrative skill, moving flexibly across structure and function, becomes especially important for the management of problem patients, those who demonstrate emotional distress and often cause parallel emotional distress in their physicians. In the management of these problems, physicians typically make many interviewing mistakes. It can be helpful for physicians to recall the principle of patient forgiveness as they strive to understand and correct ongoing or recurrent relationship problems.

CONCLUSION

This text focuses on the three core functions of the medical interview and the skills that can be used to achieve the objectives of the functions most efficiently and effectively. While the differentiation of functions, objectives, structures, and skills is somewhat arbitrary and overlapping, the ability to delineate separate tasks, understand them, and practice them contributes to achieving a higher degree of excellence in the patient encounter. This final chapter presents an integrative overview, specifying key higher-order processes and principles to guide the learner and practitioner in navigating the complex pathways between structure and function in the interview.

REFERENCES

1. Polanyi M: *Personal knowledge: towards a post-critical philosophy*, New York, 1968, Harper.
2. Elstein A, Shilman L, Sprafka S: *Medical problem solving: an analysis of clinical reasoning*, Cambridge, Mass, 1978, Cambridge University Press.
3. Kassirer JP, Gorry GA: Clinical problem solving: a behavioral analysis, *Ann Intern Med* 89:245-255, 1978.
4. Kaplan K: Hypothesis testing. In Lipkin M Jr, Putnam S, Lazare A, editors: *The medical interview: clinical care, education, and research*, New York, 1995, Springer-Verlag.
5. Johnson TM, Hardt ES, Kleinman A: Cultural factors in the medical interview. In Lipkin M Jr, Putnam S, Lazare A, editors: *The medical interview: clinical care, education, and research*, New York, 1995, Springer-Verlag.
6. Elstein AS: Psychological research on diagnostic reasoning. In Lipkin M Jr, Putnam S, Lazare A, editors: *The medical interview: clinical care, education, and research*, New York, 1995, Springer-Verlag.

7. Nurcombe B, Gallagher RM: *The clinical process in psychiatry: diagnosis and management planning,* Cambridge, Mass, 1986, Cambridge University Press.
8. Levinson W, Roter DL, Mullooly JP, et al: Physician-patient communication: the relationship with malpractice claims among primary care physicians and surgeons, *JAMA* 277(7):553-559, 1997.8

APPENDIX

1 Learning How to Interview

There are many ways to learn better interviewing skills. A great deal depends on the level of interest, experience, and motivation of the learner and the resources and organization of the learning program.

Most of the readers of this text will be medical students or teachers of medical students. This chapter discusses some of the educational approaches that have been used in learning about interviewing. Each of several modalities is presented with suggestions about how to use the techniques most effectively.

READINGS

Assigned reading, sometimes followed by class or group discussion, can be an invaluable source of knowledge about interviewing. Interested learners can benefit from an examination of many of the references cited throughout this text. Reading can provide a conceptual framework around which skills can be practiced and developed. However, there is a clear disjunction between knowledge and the skills needed to apply this knowledge. Interviewing proficiency is a skill that can be aided by knowledge, but high degrees of knowledge do not guarantee any level of skill. Skills are most appropriately developed through the other techniques described here.

Besides providing knowledge, reading about interviewing skills can help change attitudes and dispositions to behave in certain ways. Research supporting the importance of interviewing skills in patient management and advocacy by medical leaders for interview training can help develop the attitudes that are desirable to learn for future practice.

LECTURES

The strengths and weaknesses of lectures are similar to those of reading material. Knowledge can be transmitted and attitudes can be influenced through lectures, but lectures do little toward the development of psychomotor proficiencies (i.e., skills).

DEMONSTRATION

Demonstration plays a powerful role in influencing learner skills. The imitation model is one of the most natural and basic learning mechanisms in all animals. Whether the skill or desired behavior is interviewing, pottery, music, dancing, or almost anything else, demonstration provides an invaluable first step to learning. It is much easier for students to imitate what they actually see than to produce de novo what they are instructed to do through readings or lectures. However, imitation should not be taken too literally. Direct imitation may be appropriate for learning some basic skills, but learners should also feel free to adapt what they have seen to suit their own styles. This freedom is particularly important for learning higher-order skills. Complex and higher-order skills are much subtler and cannot be easily imitated. They therefore depend a great deal more on the characteristics and style of the particular doctor.

Demonstration can be accomplished in several different ways. Learners can watch videotapes of effective interviewing or observe live demonstrations by an instructor with real patients. Interviewing skills can also be effectively demonstrated by using role-play or standardized patient techniques.[1,2]

The most important part of effective demonstration is observing a model in discrete, digestible chunks. When the modeled behavior extends over a long time (more than 3 to 4 minutes) or contains an assortment of unclear behaviors, the model can serve more to confuse or dazzle than to aid the learner. A demonstration must be short enough for learners to remember what they saw, and it also must be structured to allow learners to analyze it in categories of behavior that are understandable and digestible.

PRACTICE

There is no substitute for practice. This holds true for any skill. Playing tennis, playing the piano, and performing surgery all require practice. Interviewing is the same. Interviewing can be practiced in role-play, with simulated patients, or with real patients.

Although necessary for proficiency, practice is certainly not sufficient. Just as the tennis player can develop bad habits that interfere with proficiency, so can physicians develop bad habits that interfere with their communication skills. To be maximally useful to learners, practice must be coupled with observation and feedback.

OBSERVATION AND FEEDBACK

Learners need the opportunity to obtain feedback on their performance.[3] There are numerous ways to obtain this feedback. Most commonly, teachers offer feedback on students' performance. Motivated self-learners can audiotape or videotape their interactions with patients, review these, and become their own self-critics. Alternatively, learners can solicit feedback from colleagues. In addition, learners can request feedback from actual patients. Obtaining honest feedback from patients can be difficult, but this is possible if the learner convinces the patient that he or she is sincere in the effort to obtain both positive and negative feedback.

Feedback should be obtained immediately after the designated behavior. The longer the interval between actual performance and feedback, the lower the potential for learning. Learners should be given both positive and negative (constructive) feedback. Feedback is much more useful if it is concrete and specific. Moreover, it is usually better to give positive feedback first. Learners and teachers are too quick to focus only on the negative behaviors. To help develop skills in self-observation, learners will find it useful to give their own positive and negative feedback to themselves first and then to seek feedback from other observers.

REPETITIVE PRACTICE

Once a learner has obtained feedback on performance, he or she must use this feedback in repeated efforts. Feedback often is given in learning situations without learners having the opportunity to practice the skill again and attain a more successful outcome. An opportunity for significant learning is missed if feedback is obtained without the opportunity for repetitive practice. Repeated practice under the observation of an instructor also allows the opportunity for the learner to test whether he or she has actually mastered the problem at hand. If the learner does not succeed at this repeated attempt, he or she can be given yet another opportunity to attempt to meet the challenge at hand.

When using live patients and videotape material, it may be difficult to obtain opportunities for immediate repetitive practice. After a review of live or videotaped patient interviews, spontaneous role-play techniques can be especially useful in crafting simulations that allow learners the opportunity for repetitive practice of skills that are difficult to learn.[1]

VIDEOTAPE

Videotape is an invaluable method for learners to observe their behavior with patients. Videotapes can be stopped at any point to allow for a discussion and review of specific behaviors. In addition, there is no better vehicle to discuss nonverbal communication. Both the patient's nonverbal behavior and the interviewer's nonverbal signals can be scrutinized.

Using videotape to learn interviewing has a few drawbacks. Some learners, especially those who are not skilled or confident, may be distressed by videotape-based feedback, particularly if it is given in front of their peers. Such a situation can impede learning. Videotape should be used only with some sensitivity to this issue and with some freedom of choice for the learner.

Sometimes the technology of videotape interferes with efficiency in the educational process. Ensuring that the machines are working properly, finding desired tape sections for review, and dealing with other logistical issues can take a great deal of time, time that is lost for education. When the time available for learning is limited, technology-intensive methods that take time away from actual learning should be avoided. This time might better be spent with demonstration, actual interviewing practice, role-play practice, and other "live" methods of education.

Another drawback to the use of videotape is that feedback is often delayed for a long period. The educational utility of immediate feedback may be lost when learners wait for a long time to obtain their feedback. The learner's memories of the actual event may be forgotten by the time feedback is received. Furthermore, videotape feedback is often received without providing the learner with an immediate opportunity for repeated practice.

When videotaping is used for learning interviewing, the following guidelines are suggested:

1. Sensitively negotiate the ways videotape will be used and feedback will be obtained.
2. Make sure that the equipment is working well and that valuable time is not lost with mechanical fumbling.
3. Arrange for feedback immediately or shortly after videotaping.
4. Plan for learners to use the opportunity for repetitive practice (perhaps by using role-play techniques) immediately after feedback, preferably under observation again.

STANDARDIZED PATIENTS

Standardized patients are nonpatients, often but not necessarily professional actors, who are trained to assume patient roles. Such actors and actresses can also be trained to provide students with feedback on the student's interviewing performance. Stillman and others[2,4] have used such simulated patients with great success for the teaching of interviewing and physical examination skills to medical students, house officers, and other interested learners. These simulated patients have also been used to evaluate medical students and other physicians.

When such simulators are well trained, they can repeatedly present learners with the types of patients that instructors believe to be the best training for their students. Simulated patients can be so well trained that they bear very close resemblance to actual patients. In fact, some actors actually play the roles so well that when students or house officers are "blind" to when they will interview real patients or simulated patients they may not be able to tell one from the other. However, caution is needed when standardized patients are used as teaching aids because they may not have received adequate training. When they are allowed to give independent feedback (in the absence of other instructors) to learners, their feedback may be idiosyncratic, incorrect, or even harmful to learners.

ROLE-PLAY

Standardized patients represent a special case of the more generic use of role-play techniques.[1] Role-play, however, merits a separate section in this text because in most learning situations, it has come to mean a less formalized, less structured approach to the simulation of patient roles for communication skills training.

Role-play is a versatile technique that allows instructors to focus on particular aspects of interviewing for the benefit of demonstration, practice, or feedback. Through role-play, learners can be invited to play the role of a patient, instructors can demonstrate techniques, and learners can practice basic or advanced interviewing skills.

Like videotapes, role-play exercises can be stopped frequently for feedback. Unlike videotape, a role-play exercise can be designed for immediate feedback and repetitive practice to consolidate skills. Role-play can also be used in large groups. A small role-play exercise can be constructed for demonstration in front of a large audience. The audience can then be broken into groups of two or three to practice basic skills.

The basic drawback to role-play is that learners are sometimes anxious about participating in these exercises. Instructors who have not used the techniques before may remain unconvinced of their utility and may themselves be anxious, and therefore unconvincing and ineffective. These obstacles are easily overcome. A guide for using role-play is available,[1] and interested learners and instructors can effectively use these techniques, given some modest motivation and effort. When necessary, consultation or supervision by someone who has had role-play experience can be invaluable.

MODIFIED LIVE PATIENT INTERVIEWS

There is no substitute for practicing with real patients to learn good interviewing skills. Every patient is different, and the complexities of interviewing cannot be demonstrated by using only simulated patients or role-play scenarios. Practice with live patients lends a richness and credibility to training that cannot be duplicated by other techniques.

Live patient interviewing can be modified in educationally useful ways that add to the powerful effects of the method. When observed in his or her interviews with real patients, the learner has the opportunity to benefit from immediate feedback on a variety of communication techniques.

After an interview is completed, patients can be asked to provide their feedback on the learner's performance. They can tell the learner what techniques seemed to work well and what parts did not. Learners who are curious about whether patients feel that their privacy is being invaded by quality-of-life questions can ask patients about this issue directly. Patients' responses to these kinds of inquiries are often instructive and meaningful to learners.

The rotating live patient interview is a modification of live patient interviewing that has proved useful for learners. With this technique a patient is asked to allow a group of learners to interview him or her one at a time. For example, one learner might talk to the patient for about 5 minutes. He or she can pause for feedback, with or without the patient present. Then the interview can be restarted with another learner.

Live patient interviews allow students to use repetitive practice to master techniques that require more work. For example, if one learner has talked with a patient for a few minutes and the group has stopped for feedback, the patient might be willing to repeat the same interview for purposes of learning. Patients often are pleased to help in this effort to train students to become better doctors.

SMALL GROUPS

Interviewing is best learned in groups of four to six learners. A few lectures may be useful to cover basic concepts, and some role-play may be accomplished in large groups, but close instructor feedback is invaluable for mastering key interviewing skills. A small student-to-teacher ratio allows the instructor to observe each learner and understand individual strengths and weaknesses. This effort is certainly faculty intensive, but no way has been found around this problem. Standardized patients have been used to give individualized feedback, but their usefulness is limited to the particular cases on which they have been trained. When standardized patients are allowed to give more generalized feedback, they may overstep the situations for which they have been trained. Effective learning, then, requires at least some close supervision by medical faculty.

LEARNER-CENTERED METHODS

Current educational research indicates that students may learn more effectively when they are allowed to guide their own educational efforts. This has also been called the discovery method or problem-oriented approach to education. Many exciting developments in medical education are occurring along these lines.

An educational program in communication skills lends itself well to the discovery and learner-centered process. Basic skills, however, are addressed most effectively through a creative and flexible integration of learner-centered with more traditional instructor-oriented approaches. For example, Suzuki violin, a learner-centered method for teaching basic music skills, relies greatly on independent student discovery and problem solving, but an instructor demonstrates proper finger, head, and arm positioning from the beginning. Montessori primary education, to give another learner-centered model, encourages grade school students to work independently and address topics of their own choosing at their own pace of learning. However, while encouraging this freedom, Montessori also structures the learning of basic math skills within a highly operationalized, rigid framework of materials and methods.

By analogy to the Suzuki and Montessori methods, Mack Lipkin, Jr, Craig Kaplan, and other leaders of the American Academy on Patient and Physician have pioneered approaches to learning basic interviewing skills through a flexible integration of learner- and instructor-oriented methods.[7] For example, students can and should become colleagues with their teachers at an early stage of interviewing skills training. Learners can be invited to contribute their own ideas to the goals and techniques of effective communication. A learner-centered approach repeatedly invites students to assess their level of skills and learning objectives. Furthermore, this approach suggests that learners play a role in determining with the instructor the best instructional methods for attaining their goals. Since no instructional program in interviewing can hope to attain all the objectives listed in even a basic text such as this one, instructors are encouraged to invite their students to help in determining the appropriate focus and emphasis in each instructional session, as well as the teaching methods used (e.g., live patients and role-play). The interested reader can consult relevant sources for a more detailed discussion of these topics.[5-7]

A focus on learner-centered methods should not be seen as an abdication of the instructor's responsibility to demonstrate basic techniques (such as open-ended questioning, facilitation, and reflection). Some specific interviewing techniques have been shown through research and accumulated clinical experience to be effective, and learners usually benefit from clear instruction and modeling of techniques. An analogy can be made with athletics. Consider the swing of a tennis player, usually taught through demonstration and careful imitation. However, as a tennis player advances, he or she may feel free to experiment with subtle variations of basic techniques. Similarly, basic communication skills may be modified and expanded as learners and teachers together consider the mechanism, timing, and application of their use. For all these reasons, particularly for the development of higher-order skills, learner-centered approaches can play a critical role in the development of competency in communication.

The teacher-learner relationship clearly parallels the doctor-patient relationship in several ways. In the doctor-patient relationship, there is no clearly right and wrong pattern of authority and control that is suitable for every condition and for every patient. Rather, some accept and adapt to their illness better when they are given relatively more autonomy to make decisions and to play a greater role in their overall health care. Similarly, some learners may be able to assume earlier autonomy as clinicians when they are given earlier responsibility to make decisions for their own education.

Clearly the desire or ability of patients or learners to assume more responsibility for their learning or health depends a great deal on their initial knowledge, attitudes, and skills. One common problem with encouraging patients and learners to develop confidence in their own problem-solving skills is that many are at first unwilling or unable to exercise a genuine role of autonomous decision making, with all the risks and uncertainties that this involves. In some clinical and learning situations this problem can be overcome by beginning with more structured teacher- or physician-oriented approaches. However, if the final goal is to help learners and patients achieve confidence to tackle unpredictable future problems on their own, a common educational task for both may be to move beyond early teacher- or physician-centered modes and toward patient- or learner-centered methods as the relationships unfold.

REFERENCES

1. Cohen-Cole SA: On teaching with role play. In Lipkin M Jr, Putnam S, Lazare A, editors: *The medical interview: clinical care, education, and research,* New York, 1995, Springer-Verlag.
2. Stillman P et al: Results of a survey on the use of standardized patients to teach and evaluate clinical skills, *Academic Med* 65:288-292, 1990.
3. Maguire P et al: The value of feedback in teaching interviewing skills to medical students, *Psychol Med* 8:695-704, 1978.
4. Stillman P et al: An assessment of the clinical skills of fourth-year students at four New England medical schools, *Academic Med* 65:320-326, 1990.
5. Knowles M: *The modern practice of adult education,* New York, 1980, Adult Education.

6. Burrows HS, Tamblyn RM: *Problem-based learning: an approach to medical education*, New York, 1980, Springer-Verlag.
7. Lipkin M Jr, Kaplan C, Clark W, Novack DH: Teaching medical interviewing: the Lipkin model. In Lipkin M Jr, Putnam S, Lazare A, editors: *The medical interview: clinical care, education, and research*, New York, 1995, Springer-Verlag.

APPENDIX

2 Three Functions of Effective Interviewing

Functions	Objectives	Skills
Build the relationship	Establishment of effective working relationship Patient satisfaction Increased adherence Fewer lawsuits Detection of psychiatric distress Physician satisfaction Improved physical outcome	Empathy Reflection Legitimation Support Partnership Respect
Assess the patient's problems	Accurate data collection Efficient data collection Understanding of the patient	Open-ended questions Open-to-closed cone Facilitation Checking Survey of problems Negotiation of priorities Clarification and direction Summarization Eliciting of patient's expectations Eliciting of patient's ideas about etiology Eliciting of effect of illness on patient's life

Functions	Objectives	Skills
Manage the patient's problems (education, negotiation, motivation)	Achievement of patient understanding Involvement of patient in treatment process Motivation of nonadherent patients to cooperate with treatment plan	**Education** • Eliciting of patient's ideas • Provision of basic diagnosis • Response to emotions • Checking of understanding • Provision of details • Checking of understanding **Negotiation of treatment plan** • Checking of baseline • Description of goals • Checking of understanding • Eliciting of commitment • Maintenance and relapse prevention **Motivation** • Checking of adherence • Diagnosis of problem • Response to emotions • Eliciting of commitment • Negotiation of solutions • Affirmation of intent

INDEX

J

K

N

O

P

R

S